The Rumble Within: Transportation Noise and the Public Health Crisis

Johann

Table of Contents

Chapter 3 Long-term Measurement Study of Urban Environmental Low Frequency Noise

Chapter 4   Scalable Machine Learning Approach to Classifying Transportation Noise at Two Urban Sites in Greater Boston, Massachusetts

Chapter 5   **Meteorological and Spatiotemporal Associations of Urban Environmental Noise with Ultrafine Particles**

Chapter 6   **book Summary and Conclusions**

Chapter 1

1.0   General Introduction

Chronic exposure to transportation noise from buses, trucks and rail is of increasing concern as a risk factor for population health effects. These modes of transportation are also sources of diesel exhaust emissions, a cardio-pulmonary health risk factor independent of noise. Measurement challenges have confounded how simultaneous exposure to traffic noise and traffic-related air pollution (TRAP) interact and possibly enhance each other's effect.

Despite development of noise metrics in the 1930s, ambient noise remained perceived as a "nuisance" within the practice of public health law until recently, when evaluating noise as a population-based health risk has re-invigorated the consideration of the importance of these exposures. Current transportation noise impact assessments are based on broadband A-weighted noise indicators. The U.S. Environmental Protection Agency (USEPA) recommends an average 24-hr exposure limit of 55 A-weighted decibels (dBA) to protect a majority of the public from adverse effects on health and welfare in residential areas [1]. Many studies have shown that A-weighting can underestimate the important role that low frequency noise (LFN) plays in loudness perception, annoyance, and speech intelligibility. More importantly, the de-emphasizing of LFN content by A-weighting can also lead to an underestimation of potential harm from physical and psychological effects associated with frequency content and other characteristics of sound not captured in the commonly used dBA scale. Notably, traffic noise contains much more low-frequency energy than is reflected in dBA summaries [2]. Furthermore, A-weighting is not the best metric for measuring noises with unusual spectra (i.e. – noise with extremes of frequency or with unusual spectral peaks [3].

The relationship between the noise "immission", defined as the sound heard by an observer vs. the sound emitted by a source (i.e., noise *emission*)[3] and the health effect has not been observed directly, but there is evidence supporting a causal association, linking noise exposure to an intermediate effect of physiological changes, mediated through the stress response, leading to adverse health effects [4,6]. The ability to predict direct health effects of noise requires further study to develop new metrics to account for health effects [3].

Traffic noise has been associated with various adverse health outcomes that are also linked to air pollution exposure. These included cardiovascular morbidity and mortality including hypertension and ischemic heart disease [5,6], neurocognitive development and function in children and adults [7,8], adverse birth outcomes [9], and possible metabolic outcomes such as diabetes mellitus [10].

While most of the evidence associating acute and chronic exposures to air pollution and increased hospitalizations and mortality from cardio-pulmonary diseases have been based on epidemiological studies of human exposure to Particulate Matter (PM) with an aerodynamic diameter of <10 micrometers (μm), recent studies, including the Tufts University-led Community Assessment of Freeway Exposure and Health Study (CAFEH) have focused on understanding the role of ultrafine particles (UFP) on health effects as a public health priority [11,12]. UFPs are defined as PM(0.1) or particles that are 100 nanometers or less in diameter (≤100 nm). Given their small size, UFPs contribute little to the mass of PM in ambient air, but they are the dominant contributors to total particle number (TPN). Motor vehicles, especially those powered by diesel engines, have often been cited as a leading source of ambient UFP emissions and of the resulting deleterious effects on human health [13].

Meteorological parameters – mainly wind and humidity - also impact UFP distribution and dispersion, and to some extent also affect dispersion of transportation-source sound emissions. Noise propagation is minimally sensitive to meteorological conditions in typical urban areas, as distances to road-side sensors are always very small. Nevertheless, an air temperature increase of 10°C can result in a reduction of noise emitted up to 1 dBA. Precipitation can change the spectral content of sound, as a wet road surface shifts the sound to higher frequencies [14]. The behavior of particles as influenced by meteorological conditions is complex. Smaller particles agglomerate to larger particles, their agglomeration rate depending upon particle number concentration (PNC, #/cc) which in turn can be influenced by meteorological conditions. Predictive models have been developed to estimate measured PNC adjusted for meteorological conditions for specific noise indicators [15].

Relatively few studies have sought to quantitatively disentangle the possible synergistic effects of traffic noise and TRAP [7,8,16]. The question of whether, or to what extent, the reported health-risk associations of TRAP, and specifically UFP, the smallest particles in TRAP, are confounded by traffic noise remains a gap in the existing research record. Such a gap presents problems to public authorities interested in implementing adequate abatement policies [17]. Exposure studies of cardiovascular and pulmonary endpoints implicating both noise and air pollution as mechanisms for physiological and (epidemiological) population health outcomes may require more sophisticated exposure assessments involving measurements and/or models of both variables [18]. The need for more precise exposure assessment is particularly evident for children and adolescents whose exposure can vary widely based on their time-activity patterns including time spent outdoors, at home, school, and in vehicles [19]. Field studies deploying wearable, personal monitoring devices are warranted. Furthermore, to quantify direct dual exposures to UFP and related traffic noise, a methodology to co-deploy personal sensors for noise and UFP to jointly measure real-time exposures is needed.

The objectives of this book are to evaluate co-located noise and UFP data collected in two independent studies conducted in communities impacted by traffic noise and diesel exhaust emissions. The initial study was conducted jointly in Chelsea and Roxbury, MA and involved 5 months (April 2016 – September 2016) of continuous noise and UFP sampling. The more recent study (commenced February 2018) is a National Institute of Health (NIH)-funded, National Institute of Environmental Health Sciences (NIEHS) Exploratory/Developmental Grants Phase II (R33) project in Cincinnati, OH in which wearable sensors were co-deployed to characterize personal UFP exposure. Noise exposures for adolescents enrolled in the Cincinnati Childhood Allergy and Air Pollution Study (CCAAPS) were assessed for impact of short-term and peak exposures on cardiovascular, respiratory health and other health-based outcomes. This will enable a thorough understanding of the association between transportation noise characteristics and transportation-related UFP emissions by source, which will aid in quantifying their joint impacts on human health to better inform environmental health studies and potentially help improve the effectiveness of future public policy.

1.1 Background and Significance

In 1981, the USEPA estimated that nearly 100 million people in the United States (about 45% of the population) had annual exposures to traffic noise that increased risks to human health [1]. To date, noise ranks second only after air pollution as the most important environmental exposure, according to the World Health Organization (WHO) in an assessment of six European countries [20]. Thirty years after the USEPA's 1981 traffic noise exposure estimate, updated statistics increased the estimated exposed population to at least 146 million people at potential risk of health effects due to noise in 2013 [1].

1.2 Noise Metrics and Regulatory Framework

Noise metrics pioneered in the 1930s and adopted and implemented for Governmental regulations in the 1970's have historically focused on protecting the public from hearing loss due to industrial noise exposures. Disparities in the methodology to measure and quantify noise exposure have complicated the implementation of new noise metrics in the US for health-based risk monitoring.

The common noise metric in use by USEPA is the 55-dBA L_{DN} limit designed to protect against all long-term health effects. This limit is a day–night 24-hr average noise level (L_{DN} or DNL), however the DNL metric is generally inadequate to describe the "soundscape" in quieter areas. Further complicating the use of this 24-hour averaged noise metric is the fact that, unlike a decibel as a direct, logarithmic measure of instantaneous sound pressure levels, no-one actually hears a "DNL", as it is a cumulative exposure (24-hour basis) metric [3]. From a more pragmatic point, the general public has a poor understanding of decibels or the A-weighted metric. The DNL is also a relatively insensitive measure of sleep disturbance, which is associated with increased levels of stress hormones and other health effects [21].

Although blood pressure (BP) normally decreases during sleep, people experiencing sleep fragmentation from noise disturbances have difficulty achieving a BP minima for any length of time because blood pressure rises with transient noise and heart rate increases with noise levels [22]. Decreased quality and quantity of sleep elevates cardiovascular strain, which manifests as increased BP and disruptions in cardiovascular circadian rhythms [23]. And while the temporal pattern of nighttime noise is known to influence sleep disturbance, DNL metrics do not take into account the time of night the disruptive noise occurred. Advances in technology relating to our ability to collect, store and analyze noise data prompts a reexamination of currently used metrics with the objective of developing noise metrics to better assess human health risks for both acute and chronic exposures [3].

Unlike air quality regulations, the responsibility for noise regulations lies primarily with the state and local governments in the United States since 1982. The US Congress has not seriously discussed environmental noise in > 40 years, although noise exposure remains a large public concern [1]. Historically, noise has received much higher priority in Europe than in the United States. Since the 1970s, successive Europe-wide directives have established specific noise emissions limits for road vehicles, aircraft and many types of outdoor equipment, and EU Directive 2002/49/EC harmonized noise assessment and mandated EU member states to produce strategic noise maps for large cities. Similarly laudable is Canadian effort, such as the Noise Exposure Forecast (NEF), Transport Canada (2005), which is based on effective Perceived Noise Levels (PNL) as well as the number of events. It takes into account some of the impact of the tonal components and impulsiveness of noise annoyance. WHO (2007) notes that sleep disturbance relates to L_{night} but researchers also use maximum A-weighted sound pressure levels, L_{Amax} and indoor A-weighted sound exposure levels (ASEL) to associate awakenings with noise. The Noise and Number Index (NNI), UK utilizes a metric combining Perceived Noise Level (PNL) in decibels and the number of events for aircraft noise exposure [3]. Models of transportation noise frequencies, energy and acoustic power may provide a more well-defined nexus between noise exposure and UFP in health studies. Further supporting the assertion that supplemental noise metrics should be assessed for the conduct of noise exposure studies is pioneering work done by Stevens (1955) which concludes that non-acoustical factors influence community reaction to noise. Temporal and spectral variations must also be taken into account [3].

1.3 Meteorological and Spatiotemporal Factors Effecting Noise and UFP Coincidence

Despite extensive study of spatiotemporal factors' effect on variation in transportation noise, links between transportation noise immissions and their source meteorology mediated emissions of UFP have not been well defined. In a study by Can, Rademaker, et al., 2011, predictive models were developed to estimate measured TPN adjusted for meteorological conditions for specific noise indicators ((L_{125Hz}-L_{2KHz}) = inclusive of low to medium frequency noise bands)[15]. These models have shown strong correlation (Spearman's $r = 0.62$) between measured and predicted TPN based on wind speed and wind direction. A key constraint in the development and refinement of such models is the difficulty in capturing noise frequencies that are representative of traffic sources, rather than reliance on the conventional A-weighted sound pressure levels (SPL) for model construction. Other parameters to evaluate with regard to the spatiotemporal variation in transportation noise include meteorological inversions (also a factor in UFP concentrations as the mixing layer height varies) [15], traffic intensity, vehicle type, and time of day. Key questions to answer are how does noise vary with these factors, and at what time of day are we more concerned about the exposure?

Analysis of selected data collected during the field campaign (2016) for this book in Chelsea and Roxbury, MA showed agreement between low-frequency transportation noise and high levels of UFP (measured as PNC). Under specific conditions of wind direction, wind speed and other meteorological parameters (i.e. – humidity, temperature) mean PNC levels were shown to differ by an order of magnitude or more between sampling dates based on preferential transport of UFP, yet noise intensity levels (dBA) did not increase substantially and followed the same diurnal trend. Further statistical analysis of the daily ($n = 150$) noise v. particle count data under differing wind speeds/directions is warranted for a more complete understanding of the dynamics which exist between noise and UFP correlations [24].

1.4   Traffic Noise and UFP Associations in Health Studies

Since the 2010 Traffic Review (HEI, Traffic-Related Air Pollution, Special Report 17, January 2010) there is a better appreciation that, in addition to air pollution, many other factors are associated with traffic exposure – most notably traffic noise; and that these may either confound or modify the health effects of TRAP. Yet the questions of whether, or to what extent, the reported associations of UFP in TRAP are confounded by traffic noise remain essentially uncharacterized [25].

In a recent systematic review, the correlations between long-term traffic noise and transportation-sourced air pollution were reported to cover a wide range: from 0.16 to 0.72 [16]. However, in a recent study in London, Fecht and colleagues (2016) found low correlations near major roads, suggesting that it may be possible to determine the independent effects of TRAP and traffic noise [26]. Although not focused specifically on UFP, a study in Germany (2011) suggested that separation of background PM matter concentration and traffic exposure can be achieved because traffic-related PM is only one component among many that determine urban background concentration of PM and that traffic-related PM and traffic noise follow different dispersion patterns [27].

1.5   Measurement of Joint Exposures of Noise and UFP Exposures

A possible methodology to separately measure and assess co-exposures to both noise and UFP from transportation sources involves the joint, real-time measurement of both constituents using wearable, personal exposure monitors (sensors). Challenges in measuring UFP have been limited to deploying costly (US\$20,000 -\$30,000) desktop-size devices with limited portability. Stationary sampling of UFPs has been somewhat effective, yet it fails to capture "breathing zone" or personal-scale exposures for study participants. Further challenges to measure UFP exposure in a fixed monitoring location are complicated by the high spatiotemporal variability and the physical properties of UFP which vary as a function of distance from roadway sources. For these reasons, epidemiologic studies often use empirical models to estimate UFP exposures.

Recent studies, including the Tufts University-led CAFEH study have focused on utilizing mobile monitoring techniques, with traditional UFP analyzers deployed in a mobile lab to assess and correlate ambient PNC differences between multiple monitoring platforms (central, fixed-site; short-term residential site and mobile) to compare the temporal patterns and the spatial heterogeneity of PNC and identify factors that affect correlations across the platforms. CAFEH study results suggest that combining stationary and mobile monitoring may lead to improved characterization of UFP in urban areas [28].

However, as individuals move between microenvironments throughout the day, personal exposures can be widely disparate from pollutant levels measured at fixed or mobile monitoring stations, more so from proxy measurements estimated from models. The ability to characterize personal exposures to both noise and UFP with high spatiotemporal resolution is needed. Pairing a personal UFP sensor with a personal noise exposure monitoring device developed specifically to jointly measure real-time co-exposures from common transportation sources will allow for an improved understanding of these co-exposures [19]. Two such personal monitoring devices were utilized for the NIH/NIEHS R33 study. Here, dual sensors were co-deployed to characterize personal UFP and noise exposures for adolescents enrolled in the Cincinnati Childhood Allergy and Air Pollution Study (CCAAPS) to assess the impact of short-term and peak exposures on a variety of health-based outcomes.

1.6   Aims of book

Aim 1: Measure Joint Exposures of Noise and UFP to Better Define Associations and Possible Correlations for Human Health Studies: In addition to air pollution, many other factors are associated with traffic exposure – most notably traffic noise; these may either confound or modify the health effects of TRAP, in particular UFP. Yet the questions of whether, or to what extent, the reported associations of UFP are confounded by traffic noise remain unclear. A possible methodologic approach to separately measure and assess co-exposures to both noise and UFP from transportation sources involves the joint, real-time measurement of both factors using wearable, personal exposure monitors (sensors). Aim # 1 will utilize the data sets from the Cincinnati study, in which dual sensors were co-deployed to characterize personal UFP and noise exposures for adolescent study participants and assess the impact in a pilot study of short-term and peak exposures on heart rate as an outcome. A wearable, personal noise exposure sensor was developed and validated as a prototype specifically for use in this Doctoral book.

Aim 2: Identify Appropriate Transportation Noise Analytics and Metrics for Human Health Studies: Conventional measures of noise exposure are not designed for the study of the health effects related effects from ambient noise, as these methods arise from industrial/occupational noise exposure assessment and abatement applications. Aim # 2 will address the question: What is the most appropriate measure or metric of noise exposure for ambient noise health impact studies? Aim # 2 will evaluate the use of existing health-based noise metrics, including threshold exposure metrics, and instantaneous vs. cumulative noise exposures as they relate to assessing acute vs. chronic noise exposures. From the data sets collected in Chelsea and Roxbury, MA, Aim # 2 will characterize transportation noise exposure by employing a wider range of the noise spectrum than is traditionally used. These data elements include the frequency content as the most notable feature, but will also include other features, such as, modulation, acoustic power, overtones, Doppler effects, etc. This is a more sophisticated approach than solely extracting the overall audible acoustic energy measured as A-weighted SPL. An evaluation of noise metrics (PNL, ASEL, NNI) as they relate to sleep disturbance will be examined, given the rich data sets from Boston will allow for quantification of both noise intensity and duration from varying transportation sources (e.g. – aircraft, rail, trucks) identified spectrally, and mapped to receptor sites (primarily residential) proximate to rail and roadways.

Aim 3: Evaluate Meteorological and Spatiotemporal Parameters Associated with Variations in UFP Concentrations Emitted from Transportation Sources Identified by Non-conventional Noise Metrics: The dynamic relationship between sources of transportation noise and associated UFP emissions as mediated by meteorology is not well understood. A key constraint in the development and refinement of predictive models is the difficulty in capturing noise frequencies that are representative of different traffic sources, rather than reliance on the conventional A-weighted SPL (dBA) for model construction. Other possible parameters to use in assessing the spatiotemporal variation in transportation noise include meteorological inversions, traffic intensity, vehicle type, and time of day. Aim # 2 will use the Chelsea/Roxbury data set to establish whether varying meteorological parameters (wind speed and direction, primarily) are associated with statistically significant variations in UFP concentrations emitted from the transportation sources identified by more appropriate noise metrics such as spectral analysis.

1.7   Outline of book

Chapter 1 presents a General Introduction to the book. Chapter 2 was published in Int. J. Environ. Res. Public Health 2019, 16(3), 308; https://doi.org/10.3390/ijerph16030308 and presents field study data from Cincinnati highlighting the deployment of personal sensors for real-time monitoring of

UFP and noise across microenvironments (transit, home, school), examining their effects on adolescent

heart rates. Chapter 3 was published in J Expo Sci Environ Epidemiol (2023)

https://doi.org/10.1038/s41370-023-00599-x and evaluates and recommends alternative noise exposure

metrics based on noise frequencies (Hz). It advocates for their robust utilization in health-based noise

exposure studies, challenging the prevalent dependence on conventional A-weighted decibel (dBA)

loudness metrics. Chapter 4 introduces a scalable machine learning approach for classifying

transportation noise by vehicle class, laying the foundation for potential future utilization of machine

learning in source identification. Chapter 5 utilizes multivariate regression to study how noise and

ultrafine particles vary with meteorological conditions. It presents and validates a wind-robust model,

associating low-frequency noise (<125 Hz) and UFP, factoring in the impact of wind speed on UFP

transport. Chapter 6 summarizes Chapters 1 through 5.

1.8 References and Works Cited

(1)   Hammer, M. S.; Swinburn, T. K.; Neitzel, R. L. Environmental Noise Pollution in the United
        States: Developing an Effective Public Health Response. *Environ. Health Perspect.* **2014**, *122* (2),
        115–119. https://doi.org/10.1289/ehp.1307272.
(2)   Roberts, C. Low Frequency Noise from Transportation Sources. In *Proceedings of 20th
        International Congress on Acoustics*; 2010; pp 23–27.
(3)   *Technology for a Quieter America*; National Academies Press: Washington, D.C., 2010.
        https://doi.org/10.17226/12928.
(4)   Münzel, T.; Schmidt, F. P.; Steven, S.; Herzog, J.; Daiber, A.; Sørensen, M. Environmental Noise
        and the Cardiovascular System. *Journal of the American College of Cardiology* **2018**, *71* (6), 688–
        697. https://doi.org/10.1016/j.jacc.2017.12.015.
(5)   Babisch, W. Updated Exposure-Response Relationship between Road Traffic Noise and Coronary
        Heart Diseases: A Meta-Analysis. *Noise and Health* **2014**, *16* (68), 1–9.
(6)   van Kempen, E.; Babisch, W. The Quantitative Relationship between Road Traffic Noise and
        Hypertension: A Meta-Analysis. *J Hypertens* **2012**, *30* (6), 1075–1086.
        https://doi.org/10.1097/HJH.0b013e328352ac54.
(7)   Stansfeld, S.; Berglund, B.; Clark, C.; Lopez-Barrio, I.; Fischer, P.; Ohrström, E.; Haines, M.;
        Head, J.; Hygge, S.; van Kamp, I.; et al. Aircraft and Road Traffic Noise and Children's Cognition
        and Health: A Cross-National Study. *Lancet* **2005**, *365* (9475), 1942–1949.
        https://doi.org/10.1016/S0140-6736(05)66660-3.
(8)   Tzivian, L.; Winkler, A.; Dlugaj, M.; Schikowski, T.; Vossoughi, M.; Fuks, K.; Weinmayr, G.;
        Hoffmann, B. Effect of Long-Term Outdoor Air Pollution and Noise on Cognitive and
        Psychological Functions in Adults. *Int J Hyg Environ Health* **2015**, *218* (1), 1–11.
        https://doi.org/10.1016/j.ijheh.2014.08.002.
(9)   Ristovska, G.; Laszlo, H. E.; Hansell, A. L. Reproductive Outcomes Associated with Noise
        Exposure — A Systematic Review of the Literature. *International Journal of Environmental
        Research and Public Health* **2014**, *11* (8), 7931–7952. https://doi.org/10.3390/ijerph110807931.

(10)   Dzhambov, A. M. Long-Term Noise Exposure and the Risk for Type 2 Diabetes: A Meta-Analysis. *Noise Health* **2015**, *17* (74), 23–33. https://doi.org/10.4103/1463-1741.149571.

(11)   HEI Review Panel on Ultrafine Particles. **2013.** Understanding the Health Effects of Ambient Ultrafine Particles. HEI Perspectives 3. Health Effects Institute, Boston, MA. https://www.healtheffects.org/system/files/Perspectives3.pdf

(12)   Patton, A. P.; Zamore, W.; Naumova, E. N.; Levy, J. I.; Brugge, D.; Durant, J. L. Transferability and Generalizability of Regression Models of Ultrafine Particles in Urban Neighborhoods in the Boston Area. *Environmental Science & Technology* **2015**, *49* (10), 6051–6060. https://doi.org/10.1021/es5061676.

(13)   USEPA, Office of Transportation and Air Quality, Average In-Use Emissions from Heavy Duty Trucks, 420-F08-027, Oct. **2008.**

(14)   Sandberg, U.; Ejsmont, J. A. Tyre/Road Noise Reference Book; ISBN: 978-91-631-2610-9. **2002.**

(15)   Can, A.; Rademaker, M.; Van Renterghem, T.; Mishra, V.; Van Poppel, M.; Touhafi, A.; Theunis, J.; De Baets, B.; Botteldooren, D. Correlation Analysis of Noise and Ultrafine Particle Counts in a Street Canyon. *Science of The Total Environment* **2011**, *409* (3), 564–572. https://doi.org/10.1016/j.scitotenv.2010.10.037.

(16)   Tétreault, L.-F.; Perron, S.; Smargiassi, A. Cardiovascular Health, Traffic-Related Air Pollution and Noise: Are Associations Mutually Confounded? A Systematic Review. *International Journal of Public Health* **2013**, *58* (5), 649–666. https://doi.org/10.1007/s00038-013-0489-7.

(17)   RFA-17-1-Traffic-and-Health.pdf https://www.stateofglobalair.org/system/files/RFA-17-1-Traffic-and-Health.pdf (accessed Jan 9, 2019).

(18)   Allen, R. W.; Davies, H.; Cohen, M. A.; Mallach, G.; Kaufman, J. D.; Adar, S. D. The Spatial Relationship between Traffic-Generated Air Pollution and Noise in 2 US Cities. *Environmental Research* **2009**, *109* (3), 334–342. https://doi.org/10.1016/j.envres.2008.12.006.

(19)   Ryan, P. H.; Son, S. Y.; Wolfe, C.; Lockey, J.; Brokamp, C.; LeMasters, G. A Field Application of a Personal Sensor for Ultrafine Particle Exposure in Children. *Sci Total Environ.* **2015**, *508*, 366–373. https://doi.org/10.1016/j.scitotenv.2014.11.061.

(20)   Hänninen, O.; Knol, A. B.; Jantunen, M.; Lim, T.-A.; Conrad, A.; Rappolder, M.; Carrer, P.; Fanetti, A.-C.; Kim, R.; Buekers, J.; et al. Environmental Burden of Disease in Europe: Assessing Nine Risk Factors in Six Countries. *Environmental Health Perspectives* **2014**, *122* (5), 439–446. https://doi.org/10.1289/ehp.1206154.

(21)   Joo, E. Y.; Yoon, C. W.; Koo, D. L.; Kim, D.; Hong, S. B. Adverse Effects of 24 Hours of Sleep Deprivation on Cognition and Stress Hormones. *Journal of Clinical Neurology* **2012**, *8* (2), 146. https://doi.org/10.3988/jcn.2012.8.2.146.

(22)   Haralabidis, A. S.; Dimakopoulou, K.; Vigna-Taglianti, F.; Giampaolo, M.; Borgini, A.; Dudley, M.-L.; Pershagen, G.; Bluhm, G.; Houthuijs, D.; Babisch, W.; et al. Acute Effects of Night-Time Noise Exposure on Blood Pressure in Populations Living near Airports. *Eur. Heart J.* **2008**, *29* (5), 658–664. https://doi.org/10.1093/eurheartj/ehn013.

(23)   Sforza, E.; Chapotot, F.; Lavoie, S.; Roche, F.; Pigeau, R.; Buguet, A. Heart Rate Activation during Spontaneous Arousals from Sleep: Effect of Sleep Deprivation. *Clin Neurophysiol* **2004**, *115* (11), 2442–2451. https://doi.org/10.1016/j.clinph.2004.06.002.

(24)   Leaffer, D. J.; Mailk, R.; Tracey, B.; Gute, D. M.; Hastings, A. L.; Roof, C. J.; Noel, G. J. Correlating Transportation Noise Frequencies with Ultrafine Particulate Emissions by Source: Implications for Environmental Health Studies. *Proc. Mtgs. Acoust.* **2017**, *30* (1), 040004. https://doi.org/10.1121/2.0000545.

(25)   Health Effects Institute, Special Report, Traffic-Related Air Pollution: A Critical Review of the Literature on Emissions, Exposure, and Health Effects, Boston, MA, HEI, **2010**

(26)   Fecht, D.; Hansell, A. L.; Morley, D.; Dajnak, D.; Vienneau, D.; Beevers, S.; Toledano, M. B.; Kelly, F. J.; Anderson, H. R.; Gulliver, J. Spatial and Temporal Associations of Road Traffic Noise and Air Pollution in London: Implications for Epidemiological Studies. *Environment International* **2016**, *88*, 235–242. https://doi.org/10.1016/j.envint.2015.12.001.

(27) Fuks, K.; Moebus, S.; Hertel, S.; Viehmann, A.; Nonnemacher, M.; Dragano, N.; Möhlenkamp, S.; Jakobs, H.; Kessler, C.; Erbel, R.; et al. Long-Term Urban Particulate Air Pollution, Traffic Noise, and Arterial Blood Pressure. *Environmental Health Perspectives* **2011**, *119* (12), 1706.

(28) Simon, M. C.; Hudda, N.; Naumova, E. N.; Levy, J. I.; Brugge, D.; Durant, J. L. Comparisons of Traffic-Related Ultrafine Particle Number Concentrations Measured in Two Urban Areas by Central, Residential, and Mobile Monitoring. *Atmospheric Environment* **2017**, *169*, 113–127. https://doi.org/10.1016/j.atmosenv.2017.09.003.

Chapter 2

Wearable Ultrafine Particle and Noise Monitoring Sensors Jointly Measure Personal Co-Exposures in a Pediatric Population

1. Introduction

Air pollution from traffic exhaust emissions and chronic ambient noise exposure frequently occur together in urban areas, adversely impacting population health outcomes. Epidemiological studies have linked both air pollution and noise to common adverse health outcomes such as increased blood pressure and myocardial infarction [1], and some research has shown adverse effects on pulmonary function due to the combined effects of air pollution and noise stress [2] .

Most of the evidence supporting the link between acute and chronic exposures to air pollution and increased hospitalizations and mortality from cardio-pulmonary diseases has been based on epidemiological studies of human exposure to fine particulate matter ($PM_{2.5}$). Recent studies, including the Tufts University-led Community Assessment of Freeway Exposure and Health Study (CAFEH) have focused on understanding the role of ultrafine particles (UFP) on health effects as a public health priority [3,4]. UFPs are defined as particles that are 100 nanometers or less in diameter (≤ 100 nm). Given their small size, UFPs contribute little to the mass of particulate matter in ambient air but are the dominant contributors to total particle number (TPN). In single pollutant models, UFPs were associated with incident wheezing, current asthma, lower spirometric values, and increased asthma-related emergency department visits among children [5]. Motor vehicles, especially those powered by diesel engines, have often been cited as a leading source of ambient UFP emissions and of deleterious effects on human health [6].

Traffic noise has been independently associated with various adverse health outcomes, most notably cardiovascular morbidity and mortality, including hypertension and ischemic heart disease [7,8]. Traffic noise has additionally been associated with impaired neurocognitive development and function in children and adults [9,10], reproductive failure and low birthweight [11], and diabetes mellitus as a possible metabolic outcome [12]; all of these outcomes are linked to exposure to air pollution as well. Research on noise exposure to urban cyclists in Belgium has shown that engine-related traffic noise encountered along the bicyclist's route is a valid indicator of black carbon (BC), yet BC does not correlate with noise expressed as A-weighted equivalent sound pressure levels (LAeq)[13]. The Belgian study suggests utilizing simultaneous measurements of joint noise and TRAP (BC and UFP) to identify such contrasts in exposures [14].

A-weighting of sound pressure levels is based on early work by Fletcher and Munson [15] to establish equal-loudness curves dependent on both amplitude and frequency of sound. The A-weighted sound level metric has been found to correlate well with human perception of environmental noise and is specified for sound level meters (SLM) currently used for transportation and community noise studies [16]. Current transportation noise impact assessments are usually based on broadband A-weighted noise indicator, although many studies have shown that A-weighting can underestimate the important role low frequency noise (LFN) plays in loudness perception, annoyance, and speech intelligibility. Despite this, A-weighted sound pressure levels (SPL), or dBA has continued to be the predominant measurement descriptor for noise assessment [17]. Predictive models have been developed to estimate measured TPN adjusted for meteorological conditions for specific noise indicators (L_{125Hz} -L_{2kHz} = low to med frequency noise bands) [18]. A key constraint in the development and refinement of such models is the difficulty in capturing noise frequencies that are representative of traffic sources, rather than reliance on the conventional A-weighted SPL, dBA for model construction. Measuring the spectral content of the noise exposure is necessary to achieve valid spatiotemporal models [13].

Accurately measuring personal or breathing zone exposure to air pollutants remains a significant challenge to determining their impact on human health. The need for more precise exposure assessment is particularly evident for children and adolescents whose exposure can vary widely based on their time-activity patterns, including time spent outdoors, at home, school, and in vehicles. Of particular interest is exposure assessment of microenvironments where both UFP and noise exposures are, *a priori*, expected to be elevated – e.g. in vehicles, during school commutes. This objective of this pilot field study was to jointly measure both UFP and noise exposures on a personal-scale, defined as a distance of <30cm between the sampler and the exposure point (e.g. breathing zone, ear canals) [19], using wearable monitors for both constituents.

2. Materials and Methods

To characterize personal exposures to both UFP and noise we utilized two tools, both developed and validated in laboratory settings and capable of measuring personal-scale exposures to UFP and noise with high spatiotemporal resolution. The UFP monitoring device is a Personal UFP (PUFP, Enmont, LLC) particle counter, model C200 (Figures 1(a)(b)). The PUFP C200 is a portable, water-based condensation particle counter, with particle size range 6 nm to ≥3um, particle counting range 0 to $2.0x10^5$ particles/cm^3, counting accuracy +/-10%, response time < 0.5 second and sampling frequency of 0.1-1.0 second. The PUFP sampler operates on a Li-Po battery with 3 hours of continuous operation and logs particle concentration, local time (Greenwich Mean Time, GMT). In addition, the PUFP incorporates a GPS receiver, which appends geolocation to corresponding UFP measurements. All data is recorded to an external micro SD card. The device dimensions are 7x10x13 cm and weighs 0.75 kg. Results of an initial field test, prior to this study, found the sensor to be mobile, rugged, and able to provide accurate spatiotemporal measurements of personal UFP exposure [20].

We paired the PUFP sampler with NEATVIBEwear™ (Noise Exposure, Activity-Time and Vibration wearable), a personal noise monitoring device developed by the authors (Leaffer, Doroff) that allows users to view their noise exposure levels (A-weighted decibels, dBA) and monitor time-weighted exposures (Figure 1(c)).

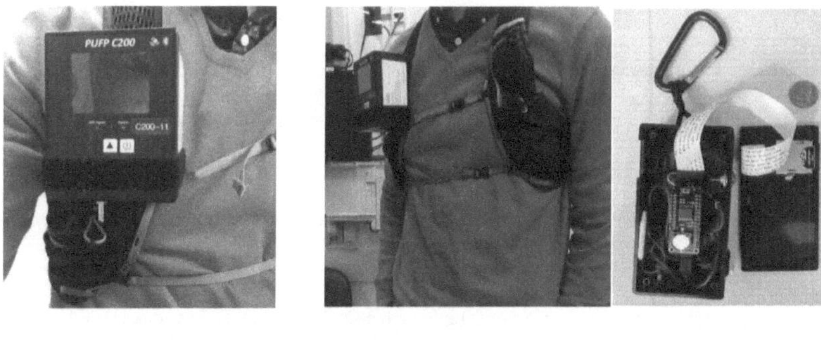

(a) **(b)** **(c)**

***Figure 1.** Photographs of PUFP C200 sampler and NEATVIBEwear personal noise exposure monitor: (**a**) and (**b**) PUFP C200 Personal UFP particle counter worn by participant; (**c**) NEATVIBEwear noise monitor internal components. The dimensions of NEATVIBEwear are 13x7x4 cm (US quarter shown for scale). NEATVIBEwear is worn by participants in the mesh pocket of the left shoulder strap (**Figure 1(b)**).*

NEATVIBEwear architecture integrates an AdaFruit® Feather M0 AdaLogger with ARM Cortex M0 processor, AdaFruit DS3231 I^2C-integrated real-time clock (RTC) and Bluetooth Low Energy (BLE) messages to the application running on an Android mobile device. The dimensions of NEATVIBEwear are 13x7x4 cm, and the device weighs 0.21 kg. NEATVIBEwear includes an on-board SD card for data capture and is optionally integrated to a smartphone to allow for easy visual access to noise exposure levels, which are also displayed on an integrated OLED 128x32 I^2C display. NEATVIBEwear incorporates an SPH0645 I2S built-in digital microphone to detect sound intensity of the microenvironment. The microphone has a working frequency range of 50 Hz to 15 kHz, a Signal to Noise Ratio of 65 dBA and Sensitivity of -29 to -23 dBFS (decibels relative to full scale), with a digital output (voltage) mapped to an instrument detection range of 50 to 110 dBA via an algorithm coded in C/C++ programming language. It should be noted that PUFP samplers generate an internal motor and pump noise of 48 dB, which is at the lower detection limit of NEATVIBEwear.

The NEATVIBEwear device was calibrated to a REED instruments model SD-4023, class 2 commercial grade SLM with a sound level generator at 94 dB and 114 dB, both at a frequency of 1 kHz. A correlation plot of NEATVIBEwear vs. REED SD-4023 is shown on Figure 2, which indicates the calibrated devices are moderately correlated (Spearman's ρ = 0.47). The correlation is based on a co-location test in which both devices monitored ambient noise in several microenvironments: in-transit (car), college classroom, and a quiet office at 1-second intervals (n = 19,532). The NEATVIBEwear internal battery is rechargeable via micro USB port and provides a functional run time of 20 hours per charge. NEATVIBEwear additionally incorporates an internal thermistor temperature sensor with a primary function to track temperature for calibration of the device's DS3231 Real Time Clock (RTC). The digital temperature sensor provides an accurate measurement (~ +/-5 degrees F) of ambient microenvironmental temperature.

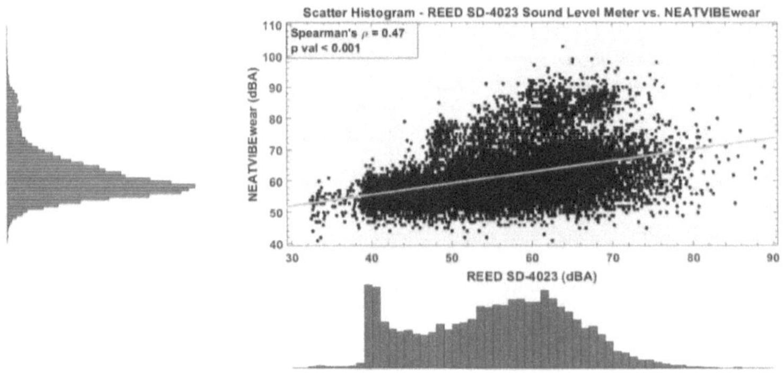

Figure 2. Correlation Plot NEATVIBEwear vs. REED SD-4023 Sound Level Meters

PUFP and NEATVIBEwear samplers were field-deployed in February 2018 on a subset of adolescent participants in Cincinnati, OH enrolled in the Ecological Momentary Assessment and Personal Particle Exposure (EcoMAPPE) Study. The study protocol was approved by the Cincinnati Children's Hospital Medical Center (CCHMC) Institutional Review Board (IRB), and all participants provided signed consent (caregivers) and assent (adolescents) prior to study participation. Briefly, participants in the EcoMAPPE Study (ages 13-17) complete two personal sampling sessions of seven consecutive days each

(14 total personal sampling periods / participant): one session during summer months and one session in winter. On each sampling day, participants wore the PUFP C200 for ~3 hours. Participants are instructed to operate the sensor and measure exposures at different times throughout the sampling period and in different environments (i.e. while at school, in transit, etc.). In addition to the PUFP C200, EcoMAPPE participants receive a study smartphone to link other sensors and apps including the PiLR Health Ecological Momentary Assessment (EMA) app. The PiLR EMA app prompts participants to answer brief questionnaires throughout the day based on time, location (e.g. proximity to home, school), and the smartphone's accelerometer.

Microenvironmental UFP exposures are assigned based on the speed and distance from participant specified locations: home (100m), schools (400m), and other (i.e. work; 400m) locations. UFP concentrations measured outside of these locations exhibiting accelerometer speeds greater than 2 m/s are categorized as occurring while in transit. Measurements that are not categorized based on location and exhibit speeds < 2 m/s are assigned to 'other.' Participants also record locations where they perceive high air pollution to be present and may upload images to give a visual depiction of their current environment. GPS data was also logged for the entirety of the sampling period using the madresGPS app; a Fitbit Charge 2 to monitor heart rate, sleep quality, and activity; and a Spirobank Smart to assess lung function. For the present analyses, a subset of EcoMAPPE participants was randomly selected to additionally wear the NEATVIBEwear monitor. The objective of this analysis is to demonstrate the usability of the NEATVIBEwear device and examine the correlation between personal noise and UFP measurements. Microenvironmental temperature exposures were also measured by NEATVIBEwear as an additional parameter of interest.

3. Results

3.1. Personal-Scale, Real-Time Monitoring of Microenvironmental UFP Exposures

A field test of the PUFP C200 sampler and NEATVIBEwear noise monitor was conducted at the beginning of the joint deployment period (February 2018) for seven study participants. Two illustrative cases are presented here as examples of co-exposures to both UFP and noise, measured on a personal scale. Participant # 300012, an adolescent female, age 13 at the time of participation in the study, wore both personal exposure monitors on February 28, 2018, a routine mid-winter, mid-week school day. To monitor and assess real-time UFP concentrations with associated changes in microenvironments, we plotted a time-series plot of UFP (measured as PNC (# particles/cc)) for the February 28th, 2018 sampling date, colored and annotated by microenvironment (i.e. while in transit, at home, other; Figure 3).

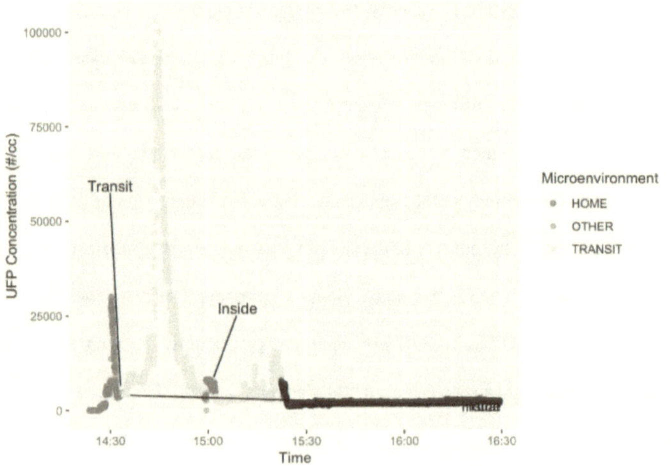

Figure 3. Plot of UFP exposure, colored by microenvironment, Participant # 300012 (02/28/18)

3.2. Data Visualization of Concurrent UFP and Noise Personal Exposure Levels

To better visualize and understand the relationship between personal exposure to UFP and concurrent noise exposure from transportation sources, we plotted time-series subplots of the participant's 1-second continuous exposure levels to both UFP and noise (dBA), with 1 minute average dBA also plotted with a

moving mean data smoothing function (MATLAB R2018a), presented in Figure 4.

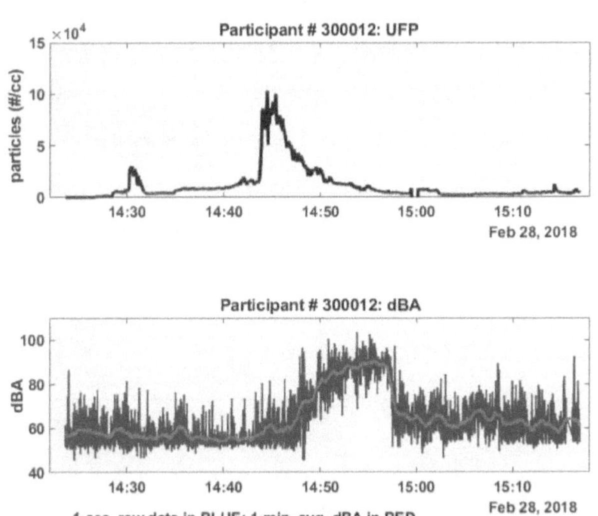

Figure 4. *Time-series subplots of PNC and Noise (dBA) Participant # 300012 – February 28, 2018*

Joint data collection for participant # 300012 from 14:25 to 15:15HRS US Eastern Standard Time

(EST) shows an increase in both UFP and noise exposures above baseline readings beginning at

approximately 14:45HRS, while the participant was in transit (Figure 3). PNC levels (Figure 4, upper plot)

increased above a baseline mean of 32.7 particles/cc (baseline standard dev. = 5.8; baseline median = 33

particles/cc) recorded during the first 3 minutes of the monitoring period to a maximum of 103,000

particles/cc at peak exposure at approximately 14:45HRS. Following peak UFP exposure, particle

concentrations decreased during the final 10 minutes of the monitoring period (15:05 to 15:15HRS) to a

post peak exposure mean of 3634 particles/cc (post-peak standard dev. = 1338; post-peak median = 3210

particles/cc), fully 2 orders of magnitude higher than the initial baseline UFP concentrations.

Concurrent noise exposures logged by NEATVIBEwear indicate that noise levels also increased during the transit (car) microenvironment for participant # 300012. NEATVIBEwear measured and recorded noise exposure levels with an in-transit mean of 51.8 dBA (in-transit standard dev. = 5.4; in-transit median = 49 dBA) during a 20-minute baseline period prior to the UFP peak, escalating gradually during and following the UFP exposure to a maximum of 98 dBA (Figure 4, lower plot). Noise levels returned to a secondary baseline with a post-peak mean of 58.2 dBA (post-peak standard dev. = 6.7; post-peak median = 58 dBA) during the final 17 minutes of the sampling period at 14:58 to 15:15HRS (Figure 3, lower plot). Descriptive statistics for participant # 300012 for the full data set of UFP exposure (PNC, particles #/cc) and noise exposure (dBA) are presented in Table 1.

Table 1. Descriptive Statistics for Participant # 300012

Feb 28, 2018[1]	PNC (#/cc)	Noise (dBA)
minimum	1	41
maximum	103000	98
mean	11765	59.3
median	5620	56
standard dev.	17342	11.8
cv [2]	1.47	0.20
skewness	2.92	1.04
kurtosis	11.5	3.11

[1] # observations, $n = 3169$; [2] cv = coefficient of variation

Figure 5 presents a scatter plot with marginal kernel density plots for $\log_{(e)}$ PNC and noise exposure grouped by microenvironment (transit, other) for participant # 300012. The scatter plot suggests that both the highest UFP concentrations and dBA levels which participant # 300012 was exposed to occurred during transit (including in car)(PNC > 30,000 particles/cc; dBA > 80). The lowest UFP concentrations (< 3000 particles #/cc) and noise levels (< 80 dBA) occurred while the participant was in other microenvironments (including inside). Given that both PNC and noise (dBA) are positively skewed, non-normal distributions (PNC skewness = 2.92; kurtosis = 11.5; dBA skewness 1.04, kurtosis = 3.11; n = 3169) (Table 1), we plotted a kernel distribution (Figure 5) since a parametric distribution cannot properly describe the data, and to avoid making assumptions about the distribution of the data.

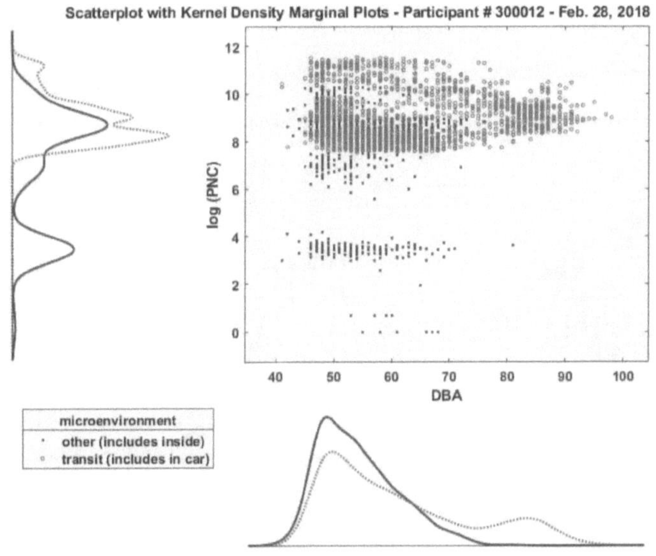

Figure 5 *Scatterplot and Kernel Density Plots of log PNC and Noise, Participant # 300012 (02/28/18)*

3.3. Heart Rate Measurements in Participants Exposed to UFP, Noise, Microenvironmental Temperature

Participants # 300012 and # 300041 were instructed to operate both the PUFP C200 and NEATVIBEwear sensors and measure exposures at different times throughout the sampling period and in different environments (i.e. while at school, in transit, etc.). A Fitbit Charge 2 was additionally distributed to both participants to monitor heart rate, sleep quality, and activity. Participant # 300012 did not wear the Fitbit during the selected monitoring date (Feb. 28, 2018). No heart-rate data was recorded for this participant for this analysis.

Participant # 300041, an adolescent male, age 16 at the time of participation in the study wore the Fitbit on two consecutive days (June 21-22, 2018). Figure 6 displays time-series plots for adolescent participant # 300041 illustrating the microenvironment in which the UFP exposures occurred. For this participant, all of the UFP exposures occurred while the participant was inside (at home), on both sampling days. While not transportation-related exposures, the time-series plots and data analysis for participant # 300041 are presented herein as illustrative examples of a home-bound participant's personal exposure regimes in comparison to the transportation-source personal exposure of participant # 300012.

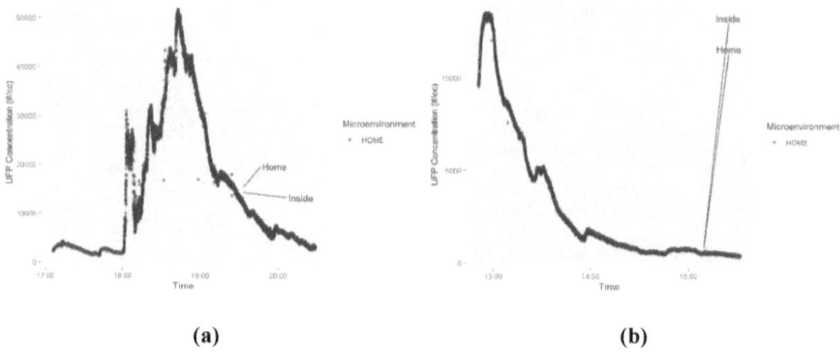

Figure 6. *Plots of UFP exposure by microenvironment, Participant # 300041 – June 21-22, 2018*

To assess and evaluate real-time microenvironmental exposures and their effects on heart-rate, we plotted time-series plots of UFP and dBA with temperature as an added parameter of interest. Figures 7 and 8 present these time-series plots for adolescent participant # 300041 during two consecutive early summer weekdays, June 21 and 22, 2018. Both sampling days recorded an elevated UFP exposure period occurring for approximately 1 hour, followed by an extended decreasing exposure period of similar or longer duration (PNC, particles #/cc, Figures 7 and 8 upper plots).

Compared to the transportation-related UFP exposures of participant # 300012, indoor (at home) UFP exposures in participant # 300041 were between 50 -85% lower. Noise exposures (dBA, Figures 7 and 8 middle plots) were within a narrow interquartile range (June 21: IQR = 8 dBA; June 22: IQR = 6 dBA) and showed little relative variability between sampling dates (June 21: CV = 0.11; June 22: CV = 0.09, Table 2). Microenvironmental temperature exposures recorded by the NEATVIBEwear internal thermistor are plotted as dotted lines in the middle subplots in Figures 7 and 8. Given the indoor exposure regimes, microenvironmental temperature readings were limited to a narrow range (Table 2).

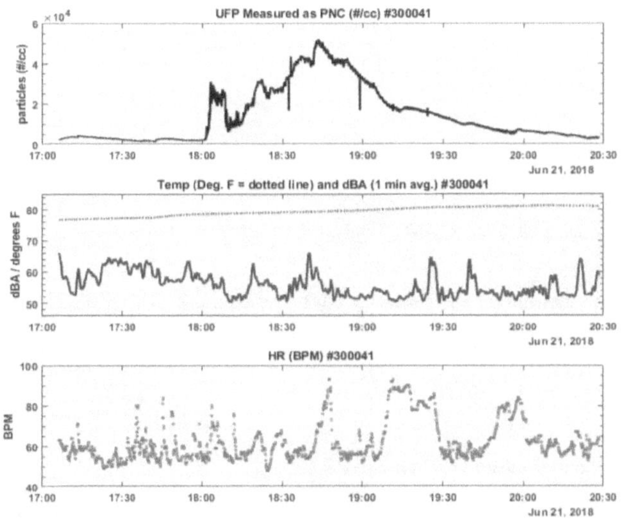

Figure 7. *Time-series subplots of PNC, Temp., dBA, Heart Rate: Participant #300041 – June 21, 2018*

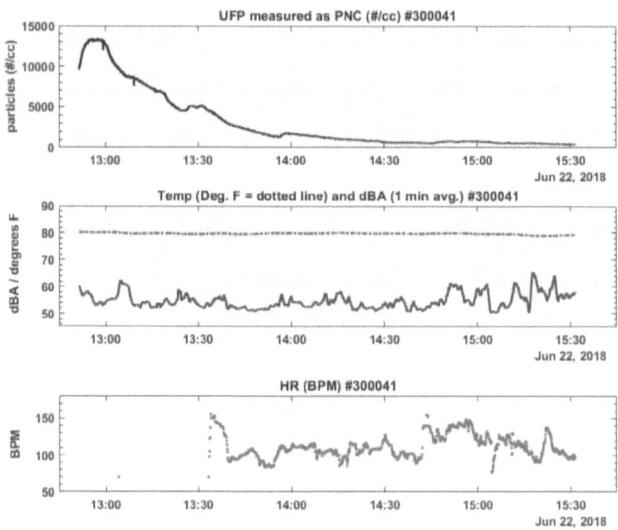

Figure 8. *Time-series subplots of PNC, Temp., dBA, Heart Rate: Participant #300041 – June 22, 2018*

Descriptive statistics for participant # 300041 UFP exposure (PNC, particles #/cc), noise exposure (dBA), microenvironmental temperature (degrees F), and heart rate (HR, beats per minute, BPM) are displayed in Table 2.

Table 2. Descriptive Statistics for Participant # 300041

Jun 21, 2018[1]	PNC (#/cc)	Noise (dBA)	Temp. (°F) [3]	Heart Rate [4]
minimum	1310	42	76.6	48
maximum	51700	93	81.2	93
mean	14444	55.7	79.3	61.7
median	8710	55	79.3	59

	PNC (#/cc)	Noise (dBA)	Temp. (°F) [3]	Heart Rate [4]
standard dev.	13572	5.9	1.4	9.3
cv	0.94	0.11	0.02	0.15

Jun 22, 2018 [2]	PNC (#/cc)	Noise (dBA)	Temp. (°F) [3]	Heart Rate [4]
minimum	354	42	78.8	70
maximum	13500	91	80.3	155
mean	3001	54.6	79.7	112
median	1200	54	79.7	109
standard dev.	3563	5.1	0.28	15.7
cv	1.2	0.09	0.004	0.14

[1] # observations, n = 12127; [2] n = 9612; [3] NEATVIBEwear microenvironmental temperature; [4] BPM

Heart-rate was measured during both sampling days (June 21-22, 2018) in participant # 300041, who wore the Fitbit device. While there was little relative heart-rate variability between monitoring dates (June 21: CV = 0.15; June 22: CV = 0.14, Table 2), the participant's heart-rate was elevated on June 22nd, although heart-rate data from 13:04 to 13:33HRS (during the decline of the UFP peak) are missing For a visual comparison of how the distribution of each covariate (UFP, noise microenvironmental temperature) varies by sampling day with the outcome variable (heart-rate), we plotted notched boxplots of each personal exposure parameter below, in Figures 9 and 10.

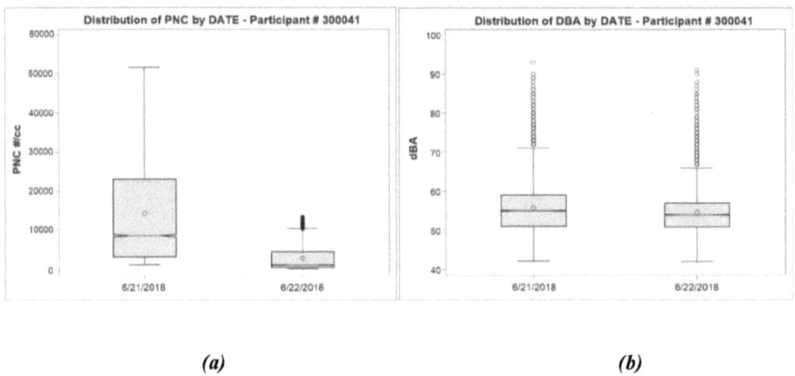

(a)   (b)

Figure 9. Boxplots of UFP (# particles/cc) and Noise (dBA) Participant #300041 – June 21-22, 2018

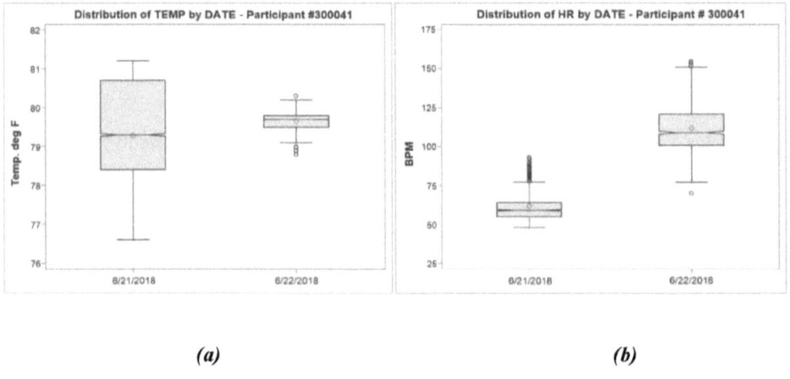

(a)   (b)

Figure 10. Boxplots of Temp. (°F) and Heart-Rate (BPM) Participant #300041 – June 21-22, 2018

4. Discussion

We found that personal-scale, microenvironmental exposure measurement with novel, wearable sensors is feasible for assessment and evaluation of co-exposures of UFP and noise on health outcomes (heart-rate). While participants in this field study proved to be cooperative in wearing the sensors, their compliance with study protocols was intermittent and to some extent beyond the control of the researchers.

However, the data collected in this field study has proven to be valuable for protocol refinement in the remainder of the study (end date = 2/2020) and will inform future personal-scale exposure assessment studies of similar design. We also found that measurement of real-time microenvironmental temperature using a wearable sensor provides an accurate measurement (~ +/-5 degrees F) of ambient microenvironmental temperature, which is useful for understanding UFP and temperature collinearity. Most exposure studies utilize average daily temperature values from fixed site meteorological records as a proxy for actual exposures, which may vary considerably as participants move between microenvironments [21]. Transportation-related air pollution (TRAP) was measured successfully here in real time using a PUFP C200 wearable sampler as particle number concentration (# particles/cc). This serves as a proxy for UFP exposure. UFP measurements were collected concurrently with noise exposure data (dBA) by NEATVIBEwear, a wearable noise monitoring device.

4.1. Interpretation of Measurements of Participants Exposed to UFP and Noise

Field study data from adolescent participant # 300012, who reported their exposure categories as "transit" or "car" and "inside" or "home" have illustrated the value and relative convenience of using wearable sensors for personal-scale monitoring of the co-exposures of UFP and noise. Our results for participant # 300012 suggest that traffic-related UFP and transportation noise exposures can be measured in real-time with current sensor technology. The UFP exposures plotted in Figure 3 (participant # 300012) are illustrative of a typical commute pattern which, in this study featured a commute from school followed by an inside or indoor exposure period. The recorded PNC measurements suggest an immediate and short-term exposure to UFP while the participant changed microenvironments (other to transit) (Figure 3).

Concurrent noise exposures logged by NEATVIBEwear (Figure 4, lower subplot) indicate that noise levels also increased during the transit (car) microenvironment for participant # 300012. There was approximately a 10 minute time-lag between peak UFP concentration (103,000 particles/cc) and peak noise exposure (98 dBA), sub-plotted on Figure 4. The elevated peak in UFP exposure might correlate with so-called "stop and go" traffic, particularly if the participant's vehicle (and PUFP sampler) was a short distance to the exhaust tailpipe of the preceding vehicle. This distance and vehicle speed could potentially be established with the GPS and accelerometer data the study participants logged while in-transit. Another possible explanation for the UFP vs. noise time lag could be that participant #300012 may have travelled behind a high UFP-emitting, diesel vehicle previous to the peak in dBA and UFP exposures peaked at a period before the vehicle increased in acceleration. We have found previously that UFP concentrations may be higher at intersections due to increased acceleration of the vehicles. The gradually increasing and elevated noise levels (Figure 4) likely correlate with a higher speed portion of the vehicle trip. This is attributed to rolling tire noise and aerodynamic noise of the vehicle itself. At a higher speed the rapid drop in UFP concentration (Figure 4) may be due to more efficient in-vehicle ventilation and longer distance to preceding vehicles [22].

Given these possible scenarios, the scatter plot of log UFP vs. noise presented in Figure 4 does not indicate a correlation between these variables for this participant but does suggest that both the highest UFP concentrations and dBA levels which participant # 300012 was exposed to occurred during transit and the lowest UFP concentrations and noise levels occurred while the participant was in other microenvironments (including inside). Establishing such a correlation is feasible in future field work using wearable sensors for personal-scale exposures across multiple participants in varying microenvironments. For more precise correlations of UFP and noise, analyzing the spectral content of the in-transit noise would be informative to verify if the low frequency content of the measurements correlates with the UFP exposure inside the vehicle. We believe that spectral analysis of selected noise peaks will demonstrate low frequency noise (250 Hz and below) to be correlated with higher UFP levels predominately from diesel exhaust emissions from large trucks and heavier gross weight vehicles, with lower UFP concentrations corresponding with high frequency noise (> 2000 Hz)[23].

4.2. Challenges in Measuring Health-Based Outcomes in Personal-Scale Exposure Studies

Jointly measuring UFP and noise exposures on a personal-scale (< 30cm between the sampler and the exposure point – i.e. breathing zone, ear canals) using wearable monitors for both UFP and noise is a feasible approach. Integration of a Fitbit device to monitor heart rate, sleep quality, and activity, and a Spirobank Smart to assess lung function complements the other wearable instruments deployed here to form a suite or set of technologies to better understand possible relationships between UFP and noise exposures and health outcomes. While measurement of personal-scale UFP is still an emerging approach, the literature cites only one study that measured exposure and health effects in children using personal UFP monitors [24]. Integration of low-cost, accurate and precise noise monitoring devices into UFP monitoring studies remains an enticing possibility to disentangle the confounding presented by these simultaneous exposures. The rate limiting step to date has been mainly one of instrumentation and measurement techniques.

An important objective of this field study was to measure health-based outcomes in adolescent participants based on exposure to real-time UFP concentrations with both noise and changes in microenvironmental temperature exposure. Based on the quality of data presented herein, microenvironmental monitoring of UFP and noise with the paired PUFP sampler and NEATVIBEwear devices (Figure 1) presents a feasible approach to collecting more fine-grained and robust exposure data than other methods such as fixed UFP monitoring sites or noise proxies to predict UFP exposures. Further, the data presentation illustrates the potential for opportunities as well as difficulties in collecting and evaluating personal-exposure, real-time monitoring data. Additionally, the data quality output from personal-scale monitoring sensors deployed in this study facilitates the ability to construct a regression-based model in which the covariates UFP, noise and microenvironmental temperature are the predictor variables and heart-rate as the outcome and is dependent on any of the predictors and/or their interaction. Such a model could be further stratified by both microenvironment of exposure and activity category.

4.3. Advantages in Measuring Real-Time Noise Exposures Using Wearable Sensors

The traditional methods of conducting noise measurement studies involve collection of noise samples manually, using professional sound level meters (SLMs) which must comply with national and international standards. The relative cost of high-grade SLM's and trained personnel required to calibrate and measure noise levels presents financial and logistical drawbacks [25]. The recent proliferation of smartphones, their constant network connectivity, the built-in GIS functionality, and numerous "apps" available for user interactivity present distinct advantages over unconnected and often bulky and expensive professional SLM instruments [26]. Yet, reliance on smartphones for sound level data collection in noise exposure studies presents its own drawbacks, such as the micro-electro-mechanical-system (MEMS) built-in microphones used in smartphones. MEMS microphones have certain limitations due to their miniature size and circuit board placement, which affect their dynamic range and signal-to-noise ratio response [27]. Another major constraint presented by the built-in microphones is the lack of access and inability to perform periodic or pre-measurement calibration. Additionally, smartphones are difficult to utilize as dedicated SLM devices in exposure studies due to the user/operator's frequent needs to answer phone calls, send and receive texts messages, run applications and other uses which decrease battery life.

NEATVIBEwear was conceived, designed and engineered to be both a stand-alone wearable noise monitoring device of low cost, with functionality to log noise exposure data to an on-board SD card for data capture and is optionally integrated to a smartphone to allow for easy visual access to noise exposure levels. A study published in the Journal of the Acoustical Society of America (JASA) suggests that using external calibrated microphones greatly improves the overall accuracy and precision of smartphone sound measurements and removes much of the variability and limitations associated with the built-in smartphone microphones [26]. By integrating an external, calibrated microphone into the NEATVIBEwear device, with flexibility to re-calibrate the microphone unlike a smartphone, we anticipate the ability to obtain measurements within ±2 dB of a SLM reference.

4.4. Limitations of This Study

A possible limitation in the use of NEATVIBEwear as a dedicated noise exposure monitoring device is the inability of the device to differentiate recorded noise patterns such as traffic noise and other sounds, including conversation, shouting, laughter or background music playing. This could potentially be addressed with a band-pass filter device that passes noise frequencies within a certain range and rejects (attenuates) frequencies outside that range, or via development of an algorithm to post-process the raw noise data to distinguish between environmental noise and the aforementioned interfering sounds. The latter approach was achieved with good results in a health study conducted in Peru in which low-cost wearable microphones were deployed on patients recovering from pulmonary tuberculosis (TB) to record and analyze coughing episodes and distinguish TB-related coughing from environmental and other background interfering noise [28].

NEATVIBEwear, in its current release, does not allow for 1/3-octave band or spectral measurements of traffic noise. This could be possible with an extended, re-engineered version of NEATVIBEwear in a follow-up (future) study or with a commercial-grade sound level meter. For validation of spatiotemporal UFP and noise models, measuring the spectral content of the noise exposure is necessary [13].

To our knowledge, this field program is the first study to integrate real-time, wearable sensors to jointly measure both UFP and noise exposure on a personal-scale with direct, real-time measurement of a health-based outcome (heart-rate) in study participants. Other strengths of this study include the ability to demonstrate direct measurement of microenvironmental temperature as a potential predictor, along with UFP and/or noise and their interactions, of heart-rate as a health-based outcome. This challenges the usual reliance on models of average daily temperature values from fixed site meteorological records as a proxy for actual exposures, which may vary considerably as participants move between microenvironments [21]. A further strength of the full prospective study, as it progresses, is the ability to network via the cloud multiple NEATVIBEwear devices worn by different participants simultaneously to produce a real-time noise exposure map of the study area and compare this with UFP readings for establishment of high exposure risk zones both spatially and temporally.

5. Conclusions

The primary objective of this field study was to deploy two novel personal sensors for measuring ultrafine particles (UFP) and noise to jointly monitor real-time exposures in microenvironments. The study focused on evaluating the feasibility of simultaneously measuring personal exposures to UFPs and noise with focus on the quality of the data and its value for interpretation. A secondary objective of this analysis was to demonstrate the usability of the NEATVIBEwear device developed for this study as an easy to deploy tool for integration into ongoing and future exposure studies where noise exposure is a parameter of interest.

This pilot field study demonstrates that both UFP and noise were feasibly measured at a personal scale for adolescent participants in different and changing microenvironments. Accurately measuring personal exposure to air pollutants, particularly UFP, remains a critical limitation to understanding their impact on human health. This field study demonstrates the ability of new tools to accurately measure personal UFP exposure, noise and temperature with high spatiotemporal resolution. Such improvements in exposure assessment are likely to benefit future applications in epidemiologic studies.

References

(1)   Munzel, T.; Gori, T.; Babisch, W.; Basner, M. Cardiovascular Effects of Environmental Noise Exposure. *European Heart Journal* **2014**, *35* (13), 829–836. https://doi.org/10.1093/eurheartj/ehu030.

(2)   Bandoli, G.; von Ehrenstein, O.; Ghosh, J. K.; Ritz, B. Synergistic Effects of Air Pollution and Psychosocial Stressors on Adolescent Lung Function. *Journal of Allergy and Clinical Immunology* **2016**, *138* (3), 918-920.e4. https://doi.org/10.1016/j.jaci.2016.04.012.

(3)   HEI Review Panel on Ultrafine Particles. 2013. Understanding the Health Effects of Ambient Ultrafine Particles. HEI Perspectives 3. Health Effects Institute, Boston, MA. https://www.healtheffects.org/system/files/Perspectives3.pdf

(4)   Brugge, D.; Patton, A. P.; Bob, A.; Reisner, E.; Lowe, L.; Bright, O.-J. M.; Durant, J. L.; Newman, J.; Zamore, W. Developing Community-Level Policy and Practice to Reduce Traffic-Related Air Pollution Exposure. *Environmental Justice* **2015**, *8* (3), 95–104. https://doi.org/10.1089/env.2015.0007.

(5)   Heinzerling, A.; Hsu, J.; Yip, F. Respiratory Health Effects of Ultrafine Particles in Children: A Literature Review. *Water Air Soil Pollut* **2015**. https://doi.org/10.1007/s11270-015-2726-6.

(6)   USEPA, Office of Transportation and Air Quality, Average In-Use Emissions from Heavy Duty Trucks, 420-F08-027, Oct. 2008.

(7)   Babisch, W. Updated Exposure-Response Relationship between Road Traffic Noise and Coronary Heart Diseases: A Meta-Analysis. *Noise and Health* **2014**, *16* (68), 1–9.

(8)   van Kempen, E.; Babisch, W. The Quantitative Relationship between Road Traffic Noise and Hypertension: A Meta-Analysis. *J Hypertens* **2012**, *30* (6), 1075–1086. https://doi.org/10.1097/HJH.0b013e328352ac54.

(9)   Stansfeld, S.; Berglund, B.; Clark, C.; Lopez-Barrio, I.; Fischer, P.; Ohrström, E.; Haines, M.; Head, J.; Hygge, S.; van Kamp, I.; et al. Aircraft and Road Traffic Noise and Children's Cognition and Health: A Cross-National Study. *Lancet* **2005**, *365* (9475), 1942–1949. https://doi.org/10.1016/S0140-6736(05)66660-3.

(10)   Tzivian, L.; Winkler, A.; Dlugaj, M.; Schikowski, T.; Vossoughi, M.; Fuks, K.; Weinmayr, G.; Hoffmann, B. Effect of Long-Term Outdoor Air Pollution and Noise on Cognitive and Psychological Functions in Adults. *Int J Hyg Environ Health* **2015**, *218* (1), 1–11. https://doi.org/10.1016/j.ijheh.2014.08.002.

(11)   Ristovska, G.; Laszlo, H. E.; Hansell, A. L. Reproductive Outcomes Associated with Noise Exposure — A Systematic Review of the Literature. *International Journal of Environmental Research and Public Health* **2014**, *11* (8), 7931–7952. https://doi.org/10.3390/ijerph110807931.

(12)   Dzhambov, A. M. Long-Term Noise Exposure and the Risk for Type 2 Diabetes: A Meta-Analysis. *Noise Health* **2015**, *17* (74), 23–33. https://doi.org/10.4103/1463-1741.149571.

(13)   Dekoninck, L.; Botteldooren, D.; Int Panis, L. An Instantaneous Spatiotemporal Model to Predict a Bicyclist's Black Carbon Exposure Based on Mobile Noise Measurements. *Atmospheric Environment* **2013**, *79*, 623–631. https://doi.org/10.1016/j.atmosenv.2013.06.054.

(14)   Dekoninck, L.; Botteldooren, D.; Panis, L. I.; Hankey, S.; Jain, G.; Karthik, S.; Marshall, J. Applicability of a Noise-Based Model to Estimate in-Traffic Exposure to Black Carbon and Particle Number Concentrations in Different Cultures. *Environment International* **2014**, *74* (2015), 89–98. https:// doi: 10.1016/j.envint.2014.10.002

(15)   Fletcher, H.; Munson, W. A. Loudness, Its Definition, Measurement and Calculation **1933,** 27. As cited in Journal of the Acoustical Society of America. Volume 5. Issue 2. https://doi: 10.1121/1.1915637

(16)   USEPA, Information on Levels of Environmental Noise Requisite to Protect Public Health and Welfare With an Adequate Margin of Safety, EPA/ONAC 550/9-74-004, March **1974.** https://nepis.epa.gov/EPA_levels_doc_1978.Pdf.

(17)   Roberts, C. Low Frequency Noise from Transportation Sources. In *Proceedings of 20th International Congress on Acoustics*; 2010; pp 23–27.

(18)   Can, A.; Rademaker, M.; Van Renterghem, T.; Mishra, V.; Van Poppel, M.; Touhafi, A.; Theunis, J.; De Baets, B.; Botteldooren, D. Correlation Analysis of Noise and Ultrafine Particle Counts in a Street Canyon. *Science of The Total Environment* **2011**, *409* (3), 564–572. https://doi.org/10.1016/j.scitotenv.2010.10.037.

(19)   Cattaneo, A.; Taronna, M.; Garramone, G.; Peruzzo, C.; Schlitt, C.; Consonni, D.; Cavallo, D. M. Comparison between Personal and Individual Exposure to Urban Air Pollutants. *Aerosol Science and Technology* **2010**, *44* (5), 370–379. https://doi.org/10.1080/02786821003662934.

(20)   Ryan, P. H.; Son, S. Y.; Wolfe, C.; Lockey, J.; Brokamp, C.; LeMasters, G. A Field Application of a Personal Sensor for Ultrafine Particle Exposure in Children. *Sci Total Environ.* **2015**, *508*, 366–373. https://doi.org/10.1016/j.scitotenv.2014.11.061.

(21)   Chung, M.; Wang, D. D.; Rizzo, A. M.; Gachette, D.; Delnord, M.; Parambi, R.; Kang, C.-M.; Brugge, D. Association of PNC, BC, and PM2.5 Measured at a Central Monitoring Site with Blood Pressure in a Predominantly Near Highway Population. *IJERPH* **2015**, *12* (3), 2765–2780. https://doi.org/10.3390/ijerph120302765.

(22)   Dekoninck, L.; Botteldooren, D.; De Coensel, B.; Int Panis, L. Spectral Noise Measurements Supply Instantaneous Traffic Information for Multidisciplinary Mobility and Traffic Related Projects. In *45th International Congress and Exposition on Noise Control Engineering (Inter-Noise 2016)*; 2016; pp 5740–5746.

(23)   Leaffer, D. J.; Mailk, R.; Tracey, B.; Gute, D. M.; Hastings, A. L.; Roof, C. J.; Noel, G. J. Correlating Transportation Noise Frequencies with Ultrafine Particulate Emissions by Source: Implications for Environmental Health Studies. *Proc. Mtgs. Acoust.* **2017**, *30* (1), 040004. https://doi.org/10.1121/2.0000545.

(24)   Buonanno, G.; Marks, G. B.; Morawska, L. Health Effects of Daily Airborne Particle Dose in Children: Direct Association between Personal Dose and Respiratory Health Effects. *Environmental Pollution* **2013**, *180*, 246–250. https://doi.org/10.1016/j.envpol.2013.05.039.

(25)   Segura-Garcia, J.; Felici-Castell, S.; Perez-Solano, J. J.; Cobos, M.; Navarro, J. M. Low-Cost Alternatives for Urban Noise Nuisance Monitoring Using Wireless Sensor Networks. *IEEE Sensors Journal* **2015**, *15* (2), 836–844. https://doi.org/10.1109/JSEN.2014.2356342.

(26)   Kardous, C. A.; Shaw, P. B. Evaluation of Smartphone Sound Measurement Applications (Apps) Using External Microphones – A Follow-up Study. *J Acoust Soc Am* **2016**, *140* (4), EL327. https://doi.org/10.1121/1.4964639.

(27)   Robinson, D. P.; Tingay, J. Comparative Study of the Performance of Smartphone-Based Sound Level Meter Apps, with and without the Application of a ½" IEC-61094-4 Working Standard Microphone, to IEC-61672 Standard Metering Equipment in the Detection of Various Problematic Workplace Noise Environments. *Inter.Noise* **2014**.

(28)   Larson, S.; Comina, G.; Gilman, R. H.; Tracey, B. H.; Bravard, M.; López, J. W. Validation of an Automated Cough Detection Algorithm for Tracking Recovery of Pulmonary Tuberculosis Patients. *PLoS ONE* **2012**, *7* (10), e46229. https://doi.org/10.1371/journal.pone.0046229.

Chapter 3

Long-term Measurement Study of Urban Environmental Low Frequency Noise

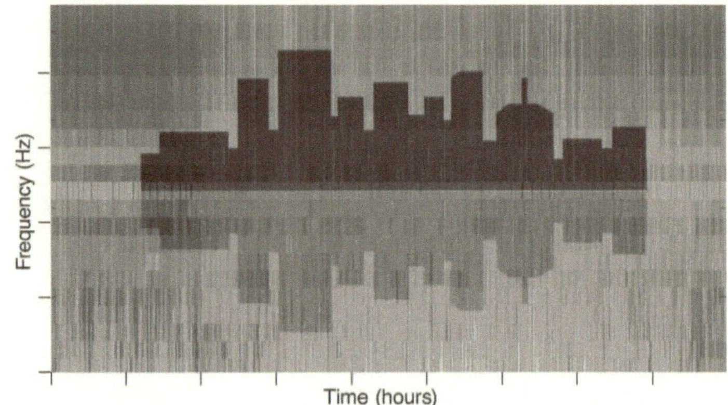

Introduction

1.0   Introduction

Urban environmental noise (UEN) is associated with a range of stress and adverse cardiovascular responses, such as elevated cortisol (Selander et al., 2009)[1], elevated blood pressure (Haralabidis et al., 2008)[2], hypertension (Bodin et al., 2009; Babisch et al., 2005)[3,4], myocardial infarction (Babisch et al., 2005; Selander et al., 2009), antihypertensive, anxiolytic, and antacid medication use (Floud et al., 2011)[5], cardiovascular related hospital admissions (Hansell et al., 2013; Correia et al., 2013)[6,7], and excess mortality (Hansell et al., 2013).

While our understanding of the biological pathways through which UEN adversely impacts health is still developing, it is known that certain components of environmental noise are more harmful than others, particularly low frequency noise (LFN<125 Hz) (Munzel, et al., 2014, 2018)[8,9]. Chronic exposure to LFN has been linked to a variety of adverse health impacts, including decreased heart rate variability (HRV) (Walker, et., al., 2016)[10], sleep disturbance, cortisol level disruption (K.P. Waye, et.al., 2003)[11]; and other stress indicators (e.g., irritability, anxiety, tiredness) (Verzini, et., al, 1999)[12]. Nonetheless, more research is needed to better measure and characterize urban LFN – specifically, how it varies temporally and spatially and when mediated by other environmental factors, such as meteorology.

The urban soundscape is dominated largely by transportation noise but in some areas it is punctuated by noise from construction and industrial activities. One of the challenges of characterizing urban environmental noise as a health risk is that metrics for characterizing, reporting, and regulating noise only address a subset of the wide range of frequencies. For example, guidelines from both the U.S. Environmental Protection Agency and the World Health Organization utilize A-weighted noise metrics, which more heavily weight frequencies between 2000 and 5000 Hz, and thereby discount lower frequencies (Branco and Alves-Pereira, 2007)[13].

A recent meta-study of LFN and health effects reinforces that the A-weighting filter is not ideal to evaluate the non-auditory effects of low-frequency noise (LFN) (Alves, et al., 2020)[14]. Ascari et al. (2014) affirm that models of A-weighted sound are not appropriate to evaluate the contribution of Low Frequency Noise (LFN, <200 Hz) to the soundscape (Ascari, et. al, 2014)[15]. De-emphasizing LFN content by A-weighting can lead to underestimation of potential harm from physical and psychological effects associated with frequency content and other characteristics of sound not captured by A-weighted metrics (K.P. Waye, 2011)[16].

Similarly, recent systematic reviews (Glazener et al; Frank, et al.)[17,18] of urban risk factors contributing to the burden of disease report attributes of UEN that were either directly measured or modeled. These skew heavily toward sound pressure levels (SPL) or the traditional dBA set of metrics, with little use of other measures of noise. In particular, there was no mention of LFN measurements in the key references reviewed (Glazener et al; Frank, et al.). Further, a recent meta-analysis by Hasegawa et al., (2022) detailing a qualitative and quantitative synthesis of the impacts of COVID-19 on soundscapes reviewed 119 studies evaluating (1) auditory perceptual change and (2) noise level change due to the COVID-19 pandemic/lockdown. In n=54 of these studies, sound level changes or noise levels were quantitatively assessed using traditional dBA metrics. Very few of the 54 studies addressed LFN or other noise frequency components [19].

To address these literature gaps, we have undertaken an investigation of UEN in which we measure LFN and noise emission spectra, A-weighted noise levels, and other environmental noise descriptors continuously for five months in two urban communities in metropolitan Boston (Massachusetts, USA). Our objectives were to (1) characterize temporal and spatial distributions in LFN in the two locations (datasets); (2) compare and contrast dBA noise metrics with LFN metrics between the two sites; and (3) assess meteorological covariate contributions to LFN.

2.0   Materials and Methods

2.1   Study Areas

We measured noise at two urban sites between April 15 and September 13, 2016. Both sites are located in Environmental Justice communities. In Massachusetts (MA), Environmental Justice communities (EJCs) are defined as block groups where median household income is less than 65% of the statewide median, more than 25% of the residents are nonwhite, or over 25% of households have no one over 14 who speaks English well (Mass DEP, 2020). EJC's generally are burdened with multiple environmental stressors (e.g., housing density, heat island effects, lack of access to green space, and noise in general) (Mass DEP, 2020) and thus serve as appropriate foci for formative inquiry into the LFN implications for urban design, city planning and public health[20].

One site was in Chelsea, a city north of Boston (**Fig. 1**). Chelsea has a population of 40,615 and a population density of 7,096/km^2, making it the second most densely populated city in Massachusetts (census, 2020). Instrumentation at the Chelsea site was atop of a 3-story building located 40 m from a busy street (approx. 7300 total VPD, Mass DOT, 2016)[21], 45 m from rail lines (67 TPD (mbta.com, 2016))[22], and 2.5 km from Logan International Airport (1100 flights/day in 2016) (Massport.com, 2016)[23].

The second site was at the USEPA Chemical Speciation Monitoring Station (EPA site code# 250250042) in Roxbury (**Fig. 1**). Roxbury is a neighborhood of Boston, with a population of 51,252 (City of Boston, 2015) [24], and a population density of 5,344/km^2. The Roxbury monitoring site is 15 m from a commercial/residential roadway (approx. 8000 total VPD, City of Boston, 2015), 6.4 km from Logan Airport and 75 m from a city bus terminal (~250 buses/day (mbta.com)).

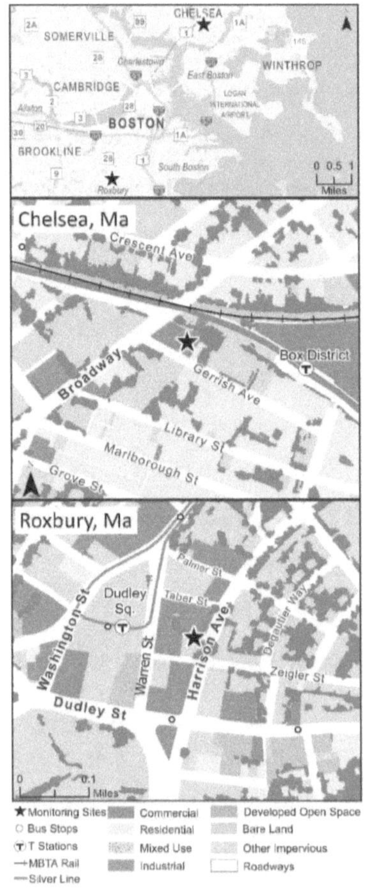

Fig. 1 Location Map of Noise Monitoring Sites

Monitoring sites are shown as black star symbols. Land use categories are illustrated by zoning type or physical features. Locations of bus stops, bus routes and rail (MBTA, T Stations) are indicated by icons.

2.2   Measurement Methods

Noise monitoring was conducted using two identical Larson Davis 831 (LD-831) Class 1 sound meters, each equipped with a preamplifier (LD-PRM831) and a G.R.A.S. 1-cm free-field, pre-polarized microphone. Microphones were mounted on 1.5-meter-high tripods fitted with outdoor windscreens and routed with 8-m microphone cables through a Roland R-05 Digital Audio Recorders. The Chelsea microphone was oriented upwards, perpendicular to its roof-mounted installation surface; the Roxbury microphone was oriented due south, towards Harrison Avenue, at a 45-degree angle to the horizontal. The sound meters measured sound pressure levels in decibels (dB) continuously over a frequency range of 6.3 Hz to 20 kHz at 1-second (s) intervals.

Meteorological data were measured at both sites with Davis VantagePro weather stations, which recorded 5-minute average measurements of wind speed, wind direction, temperature, relative humidity, barometric pressure, and rainfall.

2.3   Quality Assurance

Quality assurance (QA) methods were adapted from the *Protocol for a Sleep Study* (PARTNER, Sleep Study #25 Acoustics System, 2014)[25]. Prior to deployment, the sound meter was field-calibrated with a B&K 4231 sound level calibrator and microphone simulator to 94 dB and 114 dB at 1 Hz. Weekly calibration checks were conducted at both sites under the same protocol.

Measurements were stored on the internal memory of the sound meter and downloaded weekly. Recorded sound was field-checked and logged at both sites on randomly selected days to confirm real-time A-weighted sound pressure levels of transportation sources (trucks, trains, aircraft)(see Appendix 1. Supplementary Materials). Instrument clocks were set against the National Institute of Standards and Technology (NIST) atomic clock; clock drift was +/-0.75 s/day for the sound meter and +1.4 to +2.9 s/day for this digital audio recorder. Clock drift adjustments were addressed in the resampling of the raw noise data to synchronize with the meteorological data. Weekly field checks of the meteorology station included data downloads, battery power logs and clock resets to NIST time. Meteorological data were checked for comparability against Logan Airport, Boston historical weather records (KBOS)[26].

2.4   Data Processing

Noise metrics included both A-weighted (LA(eq), dB(A)) and C-weighted (LC(eq), nearly independent of frequency) sound energy as well as L_{DN}, L_{Night}, and L_{DEN} (see **Table 1** for definitions).

Table 1   Noise and Meteorological Data Summary Statistics

Chelsea, MA site (*n*=157 days)

Noise Parameter	Mean	STD	Median	95% Pctl	#Days (%) > Limit
L_{DN} (dBA)	65.6	1.80	65.7	68.5	157 (100%)[a]
L_{DEN} (dBA)	66.2	1.78	66.3	69.1	157 (100%)[b]
L_{NIGHT} (dBA)	58.1	1.95	58.1	61.2	157 (100%)[c]
$LA_{(eq)(24-hr)}$ (dBA)	61.9	1.85	62.2	64.7	--
$LC_{(eq)(24-hr)}$ (dBC)	72.7	2.14	72.5	76.4	--
$\Delta[LC_{(eq)} - LA_{(eq)}]$ (dB)	10.7	1.66	10.3	13.8	99 (63%)[d]
VLFN (dB)	66.2	8.71	64.6	82.6	--
LFN (dB)	68.6	4.35	69.0	75.3	--
MFN (dB)	57.9	4.08	57.8	65.0	--
HFN (dB)	55.7	3.48	55.3	61.7	--
Meteorology	**Mean**	**STD**	**Median**	**95% Pctl**	**#Days (%) > Limit**
Wind Speed (kph)	10.1	5.50	10.0	20.0	--
Wind Direction	190 (S-SSW)	--	225 (SW)	315 (NW)	--
Temperature (deg °C)	19.9	6.73	20.8	30.2	--
Humidity (%)	66.6	18.5	67	94	--
Barometer (mbar)	1015.5	6.36	1015.6	1025.2	--

Roxbury, MA site (*n*=169 days)

Noise Parameter	Mean	STD	Median	95% Pctl	#Days (%) > Limit
L_{DN} (dBA)	68.3	1.37	68.1	70.6	169 (100%)[a]

	Mean	STD	Median	95% Pctl	#Days (%) > Limit
L_{DEN} (dBA)	68.8	1.21	68.7	70.6	169 (100%)[b]
L_{NIGHT} (dBA)	60.6	12.9	61.4	63.7	169 (100%)[c]
$LA_{(eq)(24-hr)}$ (dBA)	63.7	1.08	63.6	65.7	--
$LC_{(eq)(24-hr)}$ (dBC)	73.3	0.95	73.5	74.7	--
$\Delta[LC_{(eq)} - LA_{(eq)}]$ (dB)	9.48	1.13	9.72	10.9	68 (40%)[d]
VLFN (dB)	63.2	4.42	63.5	70.1	--
LFN (dB)	71.9	3.31	72.3	76.7	--
MFN (dB)	60.4	2.34	60.0	64.8	--
HFN (dB)	58.5	2.54	58.3	62.7	--
Meteorology	**Mean**	**STD**	**Median**	**95% Pctl**	**#Days (%) > Limit**
Wind Speed (kph)	2.68	2.65	1.61	8.05	--
Wind Direction	179 (S)	--	225 (SW)	315 (NW)	--
Temperature (deg °C)	21.9	6.58	22.7	31.8	--
Humidity (%)	71.4	11.8	72.6	89.2	--
Barometer (mbar)	1015.6	5.82	1015.6	1024.8	--

In addition, unweighted (or Z-weighted, independent of frequency) 1/3-octave band readings were collected from 6.3 Hz – 20 kHz, continuously at 1-s intervals. (Goelzer et al., 2001)[27]. Average binned levels for very low frequency noise (VLFN≤20 Hz); low frequency noise (LFN, 25 – 125 Hz), medium frequency noise (MFN, 160 – 500 Hz), and high frequency noise (HFN >500Hz) were calculated with **Equation (1):**

$$Eq(1): \quad Leq(f) = \sum_{i=1}^{n} 10 * \log10(10^{(\frac{Li}{10})})$$

where n is the 1s time samples in the sampling period (24 hrs)
and Li is the 1s level determined for each frequency bin

Raw 1-s noise data were aggregated to 30-s averages for the statistical analysis per an autocorrelation algorithm designed to reduce correlations between successive 1-s samples in a vector from 0.8 to less than 0.1 with a 30-s lag time. Autocorrelation lag-time plots are found in the Supplementary Materials of this paper (Appendix 1). We additionally aggregated raw noise data and meteorological data to 1 day and 1 week for statistical analysis of data trends at longer-term levels. Aggregation of our dataset to the 1-month level (n=5 months) would not allow for sufficient statistical power for meaningful analysis of trends.

2.5   Statistical Analyses

Multivariate regression models were run on a large, two-site dataset (25E06 x 40 raw data matrix = 10^9 values) in MATLAB for meteorological predictor covariates and interactions of elevated wind speeds (75th percentile = Wind Speed HI) and wind direction to determine outcomes on LA(eq) (dBA) and frequency values (VLFN, LFN, MFN, HFN). Two-sample t-tests were conducted with MATLAB for analyses of temporal covariates on loudness and frequency Spectrograms of sound energy and boxplots of loudness data were generated using MATLAB (R2022(a); mathworks.com)[28] .

3.0 Results

We found that 1.) LFN does not follow the same seasonal trends as A-weighted dBA loudness. We observed 2.) spatial differences in both VLFN and LFN between two urban sites and 3.) determined that VLFN and LFN are statistically significant drivers of the Δ(LCeq-LAeq) >10dB metric, a widely-cited, yet infrequently tested LFN indicator.

3.1 Temporal Trends of A-Weighted Noise Measures (dBA) v. LFN

We found that A-weighted measures of loudness (LAeq) varied temporally as expected, with higher sound pressure levels (SPL) recorded during weekdays v. weekends; higher SPL during daytime hours (07:00-23:00HRS) vs. night, and higher dBA levels during rush hour periods (7a -9a; 4p -7p)[29]. LAeq varies seasonally by site, with higher SPL levels in Summer at Chelsea (v. Spring), and conversely, higher SPL levels recorded at Roxbury in Spring (v. Summer). LFN was higher in Summer (v. Spring) at both sites and followed the same temporal trends as LAeq for weekday v. weekend, day v. night and rush hour v. non rush hour.

When data were aggregated to the 1-day level, there was no statistical significance in LAeq (dBA) weekdays v. weekends at Roxbury. Seasonally, LFN did not differ significantly in Roxbury at either the 1-day or 1-week levels. Analyses of weekly-averaged loudness and noise frequencies temporally for weeks when school was in session v. not in session followed seasonal trends.

3.1.1 Two-sample t-tests

Two-sample t-tests were conducted for 30-s averaged data using MATLAB R2022(a) Statistics and Machine Learning Toolbox [mathworks.com] for analyses of temporal covariates on outcomes of loudness (SPL, as LAeq) and LFN dB values. Sensitivity analyses were run for 1-minute, 5-minute and 1-hour sample averages with no change in the significance or direction of results. Data aggregated to 1-day and 1-week did show some statistical differences v. 30-second averaged data.

Results (below) of the t-tests indicate that SPLs, measured as LAeq (dBA), are higher during weekdays v. weekends ($t(830,488)= 89.5, p=0$, 95% ci =(0.81, 0.84); higher during days v. night ($t(830,488)= 365.0$, $p=0$, 95% ci =(3.01, 3.05), and higher during rush hour periods v. non-rush hour ($t(830,488)= 74.3, p=0$, 95% ci =(0.92, 0.97) for both sites.

LFN (<125Hz) was analyzed by two-sample t-tests, indicating that LFN dB levels are higher weekdays v. weekends ($t(830,488)= 140.7, p=0$, 95% ci =(1.39, 1.43); higher during days v. night ($t(830,488)= 520.5, p=0$, 95% ci =(4.40, 4.43); higher during rush hours v. non-rush hours ($t(830,488)= 116.0, p=0$, 95% ci =(1.58, 1.64); and higher in Summer v. Spring ($t(830,488)= 67.3, p=0$, 95% ci =(0.65, 0.69) aggregated at 30-sec averages for both sites

3.1.2 Chelsea t-test Results

Results of the two sample t-tests (30-sec averaged data) for Chelsea with 95% confidence intervals (ci) around the difference in sample means are: LAeq weekday v. weekend, $t(405,497) = 106.0$, $p=0$, ci $= (1.47, 1.52)$; LAeq day v. night $t(405,497) = 359.4$, $p=0$, ci $= (4.30, 4.35)$; LFN weekday v. weekend, $t(405,497) = 91.8$, $p=0$, ci $= (1.33, 1.39)$; LFN day v. night, $t(405,497) = 359.4$, $p=0$, ci $= (4.51, 4.56)$; LAeq rush hour v. non rush hour, $t(405,497) = 159.3$, $p=0$, ci $= (2.30, 2.36)$; LFN rush hour v. non rush hour, $t(405,497) = 153.1$, $p=0$, ci $= (2.32, 2.38)$; LAeq Season (Spring) v. Season (Summer), $t(405,497) = -70.4$, $p=0$, ci $= (-1.01, -0.956)$; LFN Season (Spring) v. Season (Summer), $t(405,497) = -85.7$, $p=0$, ci $= (-1.28, -1.22)$. All Chelsea t-test results were significant at the $\alpha =0.05$ level. There was no difference in directionality or statistical significance at the 1-day level for LAeq or LFN by day of week (weekday v. weekend) or seasonally, at Chelsea nor at the 1-week level in these measures seasonally v. 30-sec aggregated data.

3.1.3 Roxbury t-test Results

Results of the two sample t-tests (30-sec averages) for Roxbury with 95% confidence intervals (ci) around the difference in sample means are: LAeq weekday v. weekend, $t(424,989) = 21.1$, $p<0.001$, ci $= (0.161, 0.194)$; LAeq day v. night, $t(424,989) = 235.2$, $p=0$, ci $= (1.78, 1.81)$; LFN day v. night, $t(424,989) = -508.3$, $p=0$, ci $= (-1.47, -1.42)$; LFN weekday v. weekend, $t(424,989) = 132.3$, $p=0$, ci $= (-4.3260, -4.2928)$; LAeq rush hour v. non rush hour, $t(424,989) = 62.5$, $p=0$, ci $= (0.832, 0.886)$; LFN rush hour v. non rush hour, $t(424,989) = 137.4$, $p=0$, ci $= (2.42, 2.49)$; LAeq Season (Spring) v. Season (Summer), $t(424,989) = 58.9$, $p<0.001$, ci $= (0.478, 0.510)$; LFN Season (Spring) v. Season (Summer), $t(424,989) = -22.3$, $p<0.001$, ci $= (-0.270, -0.227)$. All Roxbury t-test results were significant at the $\alpha =0.05$ level.

Reporting only those results where directionality and statistical significance differed at the 1-day and 1-week levels vs. 30-sec sample averages, there was no statistical significance ($p>0.05$) in 1-day averaged LAeq (dBA) weekdays v. weekends at Roxbury ($t(80)= -1.06$, $p=0.29$, 95% ci $=(-0.62, 0.19)$) and no statistical significance in 1-day averaged LFN Spring v. Summer at Roxbury ($t(80)= -0.057$, p=0.95, 95% ci =(-0.52, 0.49), nor at the 1-week level in Roxbury (t(14)= 0.67, p=0.51, 95% ci =(-0.59, 0.31).

3.2   Spatial differences in LFN between two urban sites

An analysis of SPL and noise frequencies by site shows that in addition to LFN, the MFN and HFN frequencies are higher in Roxbury (v. Chelsea, see below), with only VLFN dB levels higher in Chelsea v. Roxbury, $t(830,488) = 202.7$, $p=0$, ci = (3.02, 3.08) for data aggregated to 30-secs

3.2.1   t-test Results for Noise Frequencies by Site

We additionally tested noise metrics by site (Chelsea==0; Roxbury==1), adding VLFN, LFN, MFN and HFN with the results of two sample t-tests with 95% confidence intervals (ci) around the difference in sample means presented below. While Roxbury is the louder (higher SPL's) of the two sites (LAeq Roxbury v. Chelsea, $t(830,488) = 476.5$, $p=0$, ci = (3.56, 3.58)), a frequency analysis indicates only very low frequency noise (VLFN< 20Hz) differed at Chelsea v. Roxbury, with higher dB values of VLFN recorded at Chelsea v. Roxbury ($t(830,488) = 202.7$, $p=0$, ci = (3.02, 3.08)). For all other noise frequency bands, Roxbury recorded higher dB values than Chelsea (LFN Roxbury v. Chelsea, $t(830,488)$ = 397.4, p=0, ci = (3.35, 3.38); MFN Roxbury v. Chelsea, $t(830,488) = 336.8$, $p=0$, ci = (2.43, 2.46,); HFN Roxbury v. Chelsea, $t(830,488) = 418.3$, $p=0$, ci = (2.77, 2.80). All t-test results for noise frequencies by site were significant at the α =0.05 level. At the 1-day and 1-week levels there is no difference in directionality or statistical significance for LAeq or any of the noise frequencies by site v. 30-sec averaged data.

3.2.2   Loudness and Frequencies During School Sessions

As an additional assessment of temporal loudness and noise frequencies potentially impacting public health, we evaluated LAeq and VLFN through HFN noise frequencies for weeks when public school was in-session (school) v. not in-session (no school)(BostonPublicSchools.org) [30]. Our two-sample t-test results for school (n=10 weeks) v. no school (n=9 weeks) indicate that weekly-averaged loudness and noise frequencies followed seasonal trends for their respective measures by site, aggregated to the 1-week level. Two-sample t-test results for school v. no school are included in the Supplementary

Materials (Appendix 1).

3.2.3 Spectrograms of Acoustic Energy by Site

Full spectrum 1/3-octave band measures 6.3 Hz – 20 kHz (flat-weighted) were utilized to produce

spectrograms plotted from selective dates at each site (**Fig. 2**) to represent example weekday v. weekend

graphical time-series evaluations of noise frequencies and acoustic power. Spectrograms suggest that the

acoustic power is predominantly <160 Hz at both sites, with VLFN dominating the soundscape in

Chelsea, and Roxbury spectra showing less LFN energy on a typical, non-holiday weekend v. weekday

during traffic commuting hours. Example spectra are plotted below for days during which wind speeds

(WS) were low (<1 std below mean WS) to minimize microphone wind noise artifacts.

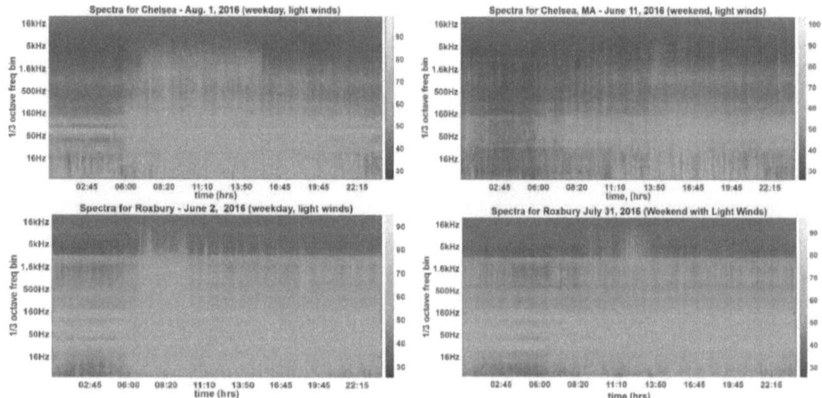

Fig. 2 Example Spectrograms for Low-Wind Conditions.

Left panels (upper and lower) illustrate example 1/3-octave frequency band noise spectra (6.3Hz –20kHz)
for weekdays; right panels (upper and lower) for weekends, collected on days with wind speed <1 std.
below mean (kph). Color bars (on right) represent acoustic power/frequency (dB/Hz).

3.2.4 1/3-octave Band Spectra

Boxplots of 1/3-octave band spectra for the full five-month time series of data (1-s raw data

samples) are presented in **Fig. 3**, and display the distributions of flat-weighted, average sound pressure

levels across the following octave bands: very low frequency noise (VLFN), or infrasound <= 20Hz; low frequency noise (LFN) 25 -125Hz, medium frequency noise (MFN) 160Hz -500Hz, and high frequency

noise (HFN) > 500Hz – 20kHz. Overall, the highest median dB frequency was 31.5 Hz Roxbury and

63Hz in Chelsea (both, 65 dB), indicating LFN is prevalent in the urban soundscape at these sites.

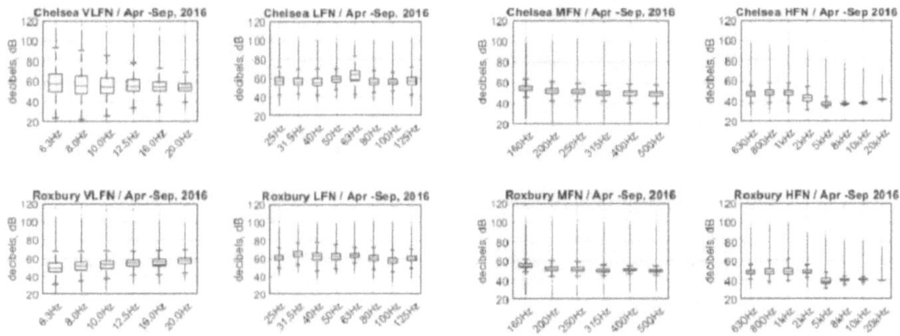

Fig. 3 Boxplots of 1/3-Octave Band dB Levels.
Distributions of 1/3-octave frequency ranges for both sites are shown across the full noise spectrum from
very low frequency (VLFN), low frequency (LFN), medium frequency (MFN) and high frequency (HFN)
noise. Boxes illustrate the median (center line of box), interquartile range (IQR), maximum and minimum
dB levels (whiskers) and outliers (vertical lines).

3.3   VLFN and LFN contributions to Δ(LCeq-LAeq)

LCeq (nearly independent of frequency) minus LAeq, (LCeq-LAeq) >10dB, an accepted and

widely-cited indicator of LFN (WHO, 1999; Roberts, 2004)[31][32], is moderate to highly correlated to

LFN and VLFN (0.36 to 0.57, respectively) and negatively correlated to MFN and HFN (-0.14 to -0.54)

in the dataset.   Covariate correlations indicate that LA(eq) itself is highly correlated (r=0.77 to 0.98) to

MFN and HFN; and moderately correlated (r=0.30 to 0.48) to LFN and VLFN. At the 1-day data

aggregation level, LCeq-LAeq remains highly correlated to VLFN (r=0.60) and remains moderately

negatively correlated to MFN and HFN ranging -0.25 to –0.30.

Our dataset shows 63% of study days in Chelsea and 40% of study days in Roxbury as having

LCeq-LAeq => 10dB (**Table 1**), which underscores the predominance of LFN transportation sources at

the Chelsea site (aircraft, rail in particular). We found that, when stratified by site (Chelsea==0;

Roxbury==1), VLFN and LFN were significant contributors to LCeq-LAeq => 10dB in Chelsea (VLFN:

$\beta = 0.175$; 95% CI: 0.134, 0.216)(LFN: $\beta = 0.442$; 95% CI: 0.319, 0.565), whereas MFN and HFN were

not significant ($p>0.05$; 95% CI's contained zero). Results differed in Roxbury, with only LFN and HFN

significantly contributing to LCeq-LAeq => 10dB (LFN: $\beta = 0.353$; 95% CI: 0.202, 0.504)(HFN: $\beta = $ -

0.335; 95% CI: -0.496, -0.174). VLFN ($\beta = -0.006$; 95% CI: -0.56, 0.04) and MFN ($\beta = -0.069$; 95% CI:

-0.218, 0.081) contributions to LCeq-LAeq => 10dB in Roxbury were not significant. For data

aggregated to the 1-day level, taken together for both sites, only VLFN and LFN were significant and

positive contributors to LCeq-LAeq => 10dB: VLFN ($\beta = 0.202$; 95% CI: 0.158, 0.2463) and LFN ($\beta = $

0.329; 95% CI: 0.124, 0.535). MFN and HFN were not significant ($p>0.05$; 95% CI's contained zero).

Regression model plots for noise frequency contributions to LCeq-LAeq are found in the Supplementary

Materials of this paper (Appendix 1).

3.4   Assessment of meteorological covariate contributions to LFN

3.4.1   Regression Modeling Results

We ran multivariate regression models in MATLAB for meteorological predictor covariates and

interactions of elevated wind speeds (75% percentile = Wind Speed HI) and direction to determine

outcomes on LAeq (dBA) and frequency dB values (VLFN, LFN, MFN, HFN). **Table 2** presents

coefficients (β, 95% ci) from the model output for Chelsea; **Table 3** presents similar model output for

Roxbury.

Table 2 Chelsea Multivariate Regression Model Coefficients (β, 95% ci) for Noise and Meteorology

Determinant	$\Delta[LC_{(eq)}\text{-}LA_{(eq)}]$=>10dB	LA_{eq}	VLFN	LFN	MFN	HFN
VLFN	0.175	0.183	--			
	(0.134, 0.216)	(0.181, 0.184)				
LFN	0.442	0.744		--		
	(0.319, 0.565)	(0.743, 0.746)				
MFN	-0.051	0.944			--	
	(-0.213, 0.111) [a]	(0.943, 0.945)				

	LA$_{eq}$	VLFN	LFN	MFN	HFN
HFN	-0.143 (-0.327, 0.041)[a]	1.177 (1.176, 1.177)			--
Meteorology:	**LA$_{eq}$**	**VLFN**	**LFN**	**MFN**	**HFN**
Temperature (°C)	0.248 (0.246, 0.250)	0.087 (0.083, 0.092)	0.252 (0.250, 0.254)	0.221 (0.219, 0.223)	0.207 (0.205, 0.208)
Humidity (%)	-0.057 (-0.058, -0.057)	-0.120 (-0.121, -0.118)	-0.064 (-0.064, -0.063)	-0.055 (-0.056, -0.054)	-0.048 (-0.049, -0.048)
Barometer (mbar)	-0.072 (-0.074, -0.069)	-0.231 (-0.236, -0.227)	-0.083 (-0.085, -0.081)	-0.065 (-0.067, -0.063)	-0.063 (-0.064, -0.061)
Wind Speed (WS)_HI [b]	1.989 (1.961, 2.018)	12.535 (12.488, 12.582)	2.889 (2.860, 2.918)	1.833 (1.805, 1.861)	1.610 (1.587, 1.634)
Wind Direction N	-0.205 (-0.344 , -0.066)	1.844 (1.559, 2.129)	-1.149 (-1.295, -1.003)	-0.785 (-0.922, -0.649)	0.134 (0.018, 0.251)
NE	-1.004 (-1.136, -0.873)	3.517 (3.248, 3.787)	-1.328 (-1.466, -1.190)	-1.508 (-1.637, -1.379)	-0.564 (-0.674, -0.454)
E	0.910 (0.792, 1.028)	6.293 (6.051, 6.535)	1.070 (0.946, 1.194)	0.937 (0.821, 1.052)	0.609 (0.511, 0.708)
SE	0.636 (0.512, 0.759)	1.901 (1.648, 2.154)	0.168 (0.039, 0.298)	0.658 (0.537, 0.779)	0.484 (0.380, 0.587)
S	ND [c]	ND [c]	ND [c]	ND [c]	ND [c]
SW	0.981 (0.863, 1.099)	4.191 (3.949, 4.433)	0.653 (0.529, 0.777)	0.666 (0.550, 0.781)	0.927 (0.828, 1.026)
W	0.756 (0.638, 0.874)	5.510 (5.268, 5.753)	0.379 (0.255, 0.503)	0.336 (0.221, 0.452)	0.850 (0.751, 0.949)
NW	2.322 (2.200, 2.444)	3.349 (3.100, 3.598)	1.466 (1.339, 1.593)	1.615 (1.496, 1.734)	2.152 (2.050, 2.253)
Wind Interactions:	**LA$_{eq}$**	**VLFN**	**LFN**	**MFN**	**HFN**

WS_HI:N	1.468	10.904	1.598	1.234	1.346
	(1.220, 1.717)	(10.508, 11.300)	(1.342, 1.853)	(0.990, 1.479)	(1.138, 1.554)
WS_HI:NE	0.289	15.814	2.050	-0.375	0.223
	(0.150, 0.428)	(15.592, 16.036)	(1.907, 2.193)	(-0.512, -0.238)	(0.107, 0.340)
WS_HI:E	1.307	12.099	2.700	1.455	0.823
	(1.246, 1.368)	(12.002, 12.196)	(2.637, 2.762)	(1.395, 1.515)	(0.772, 0.874)
WS_HI:SE	1.769	9.984	2.487	2.247	1.173
	(1.649, 1.889)	(9.792, 10.175)	(2.364, 2.611)	(2.129, 2.365)	(1.073, 1.273)
WS_HI:S	2.298	7.594	3.153	2.172	1.842
	(1.945, 2.652)	(7.031, 8.157)	(2.789, 3.516)	(1.824, 2.520)	(1.547, 2.138)
WS_HI:SW	2.493	9.675	2.996	2.227	2.108
	(2.425, 2.561)	(9.566, 9.784)	(2.926, 3.066)	(2.160, 2.294)	(2.050, 2.165)
WS_HI:W	2.276	14.053	2.998	1.982	2.029
	(2.207, 2.346)	(13.943, 14.163)	(2.927, 3.069)	(1.914, 2.050)	(1.971, 2.087)
WS_HI:NW	4.379	11.650	4.481	3.795	3.774
	(4.268, 4.489)	(11.475, 11.826)	(4.368, 4.594)	(3.686, 3.903)	(3.682, 3.866)

(a) p-val >0.05
(b) Wind Speed HI (WS_HI) = 75% percentile (kph)
(c) ND = No data

Table 3

ROXBURY - Multivariate Regression Model Coefficients (β, 95% ci) for Noise and Meteorological Factors

Determinant	$\Delta[LC_{(eq)}-LA_{(eq)}]=>10dB$	LA_{eq}	VLFN	LFN	MFN	HFN
VLFN	-0.006	0.233	--			
	(-0.560, 0.044) [a]	(0.231, 0.234)				
LFN	0.353	0.406		--		
	(0.202, 0.504)	(0.405, 0.408)				
MFN	-0.068	0.844			--	
	(-0.218, 0.081) [a]	(0.842, 0.846)				
HFN	-0.335	0.968				--

	LA$_{eq}$	VLFN	LFN	MFN	HFN
	(-0.496, - 0.174)	(0.967, 0.969)			
Meteorology:	**LA$_{eq}$**	**VLFN**	**LFN**	**MFN**	**HFN**
Temperature (°C)	-0.022	0.106	0.114	-0.001 [a]	-0.035
	(-0.023, -0.020)	(0.103, 0.108)	(0.112, 0.116)	(-0.002, 0.001)	(-0.036, -0.033)
Humidity (%)	-0.006	-0.063	-0.055	-0.014	0.001
	(-0.007 -0.006)	(-0.063, -0.062)	(-0.055, -0.054)	(-0.014, -0.013)	(0.001, 0.002)
Barometer (mbar)	-0.005	-0.078	0.003	-0.006	-0.008
	(-0.006, -0.003)	(-0.081, -0.076)	(0.001, 0.004)	(-0.007, -0.004)	(-0.009, -0.006)
Wind Speed (WS)_HI [b]	0.435	3.136	1.291	0.561	0.354
	(0.418, 0.451)	(3.108, 3.164)	(1.269, 1.313)	(0.545, 0.576)	(0.337, 0.371)
Wind Direction N	-0.343	0.558	-0.345	0.358	-0.493
	(-0.469, -0.217)	(0.349, 0.768)	(-0.509, -0.181)	(0.237, 0.479)	(-0.620, -0.365)
NE	-0.479	1.025	-0.647	-0.050 [a]	-0.454
	(-0.578, -0.381)	(0.862, 1.188)	(-0.775, -0.520)	(-0.144, 0.044)	(-0.553, -0.355)
E	-0.530	0.230	-0.468	0.000 [a]	-0.486
	(-0.635, -0.424)	(0.054, 0.405)	(-0.605, -0.331)	(-0.102, 0.101)	(-0.593, -0.379)
SE	-0.551	0.146 [a]	-0.165 [a]	-0.063 [a]	-0.586
	(-0.680, -0.423)	(-0.067, 0.360)	(-0.332, 0.002)	(-0.187, 0.060)	(-0.716, -0.456)
S	-0.561	-0.047 [a]	-0.667	-0.124	-0.588
	(-0.677 -0.445)	(-0.240, 0.146)	(-0.819, -0.516)	(-0.236, -0.013)	(-0.706, -0.470)
SW	-1.197	-0.257	-1.560	-0.805	-1.173
	(-1.293, -1.102)	(-0.416, -0.099)	(-1.684, -1.436)	(-0.897, -0.714)	(-1.269, -1.076)
W	-0.900	0.849	-0.849	-0.289	-0.992
	(-1.000, -0.800)	(0.683, 1.016)	(-0.980, -0.719)	(-0.386, -0.193)	(-1.094, -0.891)
NW	-0.799	0.800	-0.899	-0.094 [a]	-0.903
	(-0.903, -0.695)	(0.627, 0.972)	(-1.034, -0.764)	(-0.194, 0.005)	(-1.008, -0.798)
Wind Interactions:	**LA$_{eq}$**	**VLFN**	**LFN**	**MFN**	**HFN**
WS_HI:N	0.672	3.290	1.315	0.611	0.483

	(0.499, 0.845)	(3.022, 3.558)	(1.091, 1.539)	(0.445, 0.777)	(0.308, 0.658)
WS_HI:NE	0.913	3.646	1.213	0.952	0.869
	(0.868, 0.957)	(3.576, 3.715)	(1.155, 1.271)	(0.909, 0.995)	(0.823, 0.914)
WS_HI:E	1.261	3.029	1.387	1.281	1.214
	(1.136, 1.386)	(2.836, 3.223)	(1.225, 1.549)	(1.161, 1.401)	(1.088, 1.341)
WS_HI:SE	1.874	3.287	2.165	2.401	1.633
	(1.561, 2.187)	(2.802, 3.772)	(1.759, 2.571)	(2.100, 2.701)	(1.315, 1.950)
WS_HI:S	1.208	2.821	1.504	1.645	1.030
	(1.025, 1.390)	(2.539, 3.104)	(1.267, 1.740)	(1.470, 1.820)	(0.845, 1.215)
WS_HI:SW	0.023 [a]	2.775	0.941	0.080	-0.062
	(-0.007, 0.052)	(2.730, 2.820)	(0.903, 0.979)	(0.052, 0.108)	(-0.092, -0.033)
WS_HI:W	0.576	4.145	1.646	0.765	0.407
	(0.516, 0.637)	(4.052, 4.239)	(1.568, 1.724)	(0.707, 0.823)	(0.346, 0.469)
WS_HI:NW	0.724	4.867	1.677	0.870	0.561
	(0.649, 0.799)	(4.750, 4.983)	(1.580, 1.775)	(0.797, 0.942)	(0.484, 0.637)

(a) p-val >0.05
(b) Wind Speed HI (WS_HI) = 75% percentile (kph)

With few exceptions (*p-vals>0.05* indicated in **Tables 2, 3**), all five meteorological covariates (temperature, humidity, barometric pressure, wind speed and direction) were statistically significant predictors of noise outcomes of LAeq and noise frequency dB levels (VLFN, LFN, MFN and HFN). Though LAeq and frequency bands (VLFN, LFN, MFN, HFN) are weakly or negligibly correlated ($r<0.28$) to meteorological covariates. A covariate correlation matrix is presented in this paper's Supplementary Materials (Appendix 1).

As relative humidity (%) and barometric pressure (millibars Hg, (mbar)) increased, noise levels decreased marginally at both sites. Increases in temperature (deg °C) resulted in minimal positive increases in LAeq and noise frequency dB levels at Chelsea, and negligible or insignificant positive or negative effects on LAeq and noise frequency dB levels in Roxbury. We also aggregated meteorological data to the 1-day and 1-week levels to assess any change in the direction of effects and their significance

on loudness and noise frequencies. The results are presented in Appendix , Supplementary Tables 2S, 3S.

3.4.2   Wind Direction Effects on Loudness and Frequency

Wind speed and wind direction effects varied considerably by site and by outcome variables. At

Chelsea, wind directions from the North and Northeast (0 - 45 deg) were associated with reduced LAeq

dBA levels and reduced noise frequency dB levels, with exception of VLFN levels, which increased 1.8 –

3.5 dB during N to E sector wind directions. Wind directions from other compass bearings resulted in a

positive increase to all LAeq and noise frequency dB values in Chelsea, with VLFN most affected (1.9 –

6.3 dB). Roxbury wind direction from the SE had no significant effects on noise frequency levels for

VLFN, LFN, and MFN. Additionally, winds from the NW, NE and E sectors also had no significant

effects on MFN in Roxbury. Winds from other sectors had mostly negative but negligible effects on

LAeq and other noise frequencies, with the exception of VLFN, where wind direction imparted a slightly

positive affect (increased dB), when significant. The Nubian Station (formerly Dudley Square) MBTA

bus terminal is located 100 m. WNW of the Roxbury site. When aggregated to the 1-day level, the only

significant wind direction effects on noise outcomes were SSE winds at Chelsea (wind impact sector from

Logan Airport) negatively effecting MFN (β = -2.90; 95% CI: -5.64, -0.164) and westerly (W) winds at

Roxbury (wind impact sector from the bus station) positively effecting LFN (β = 2.51; 95% CI: 0.325,

4.69). At the 1-week data averaging level, no wind directions were significant predictors of any noise

frequency or loudness at either site.

3.4.3   Interactions of Wind Speed and Direction

Wind speeds greater than the 75th percentile (Wind Speed HI) were modeled for their effects and

interactions with wind direction on noise parameters. The most significant effect of high wind speeds,

irrespective of wind direction, were on VLFN, with a substantial increase (β = 12.5; 95% CI: 12.49,

12.58) in VLFN dB levels during high wind speeds at Chelsea; and to a lesser degree (β = 3.1; 95% CI:

3.11, 3.16) at Roxbury. LFN was minimally affected by high wind speeds at either site.

Interactions of wind direction and Wind Speed HI (**Tables 2, 3**) all imparted a positive effect (increased dB) on all noise measures and frequencies for both sites, with one exception: SW winds at elevated speeds (75% percentile) in Roxbury were not significant for its effects on LAeq and had a slight negative effect on HFN. Wind interactions had the greatest positive effects on VLFN at both sites, with a notably higher increase in VLFN dB levels (4.1 -4.9 dB) from the direction of the Nubian Station bus terminal v. other wind sector directions in Roxbury. At the 1-day data aggregation level, wind interactions had the greatest positive effects on VLFN in Chelsea and Roxbury. At the 1-week data aggregation level no interactions of wind direction and Wind Speed HI were significant (p>0.05).

Wind roses (plots) for LAeq and noise frequencies are found in the Supplementary Materials section of this paper (Appendix 1). The results of regression models for data aggregated to 1-day and 1-week are presented in Supplementary Tables 2S and 3S (Appendix 1).

4.0   Discussion

4.1   Main Findings

This study measured five months of urban environmental noise (UEN) at two urban sites located in densely populated Environmental Justice communities (EJCs) in Greater Boston, Massachusetts, burdened by close proximity to bus, rail, aircraft routes. A key aim of the study was to characterize the low frequency (LFN<125Hz) components of UEN, specifically, how it varies temporally and when mediated by other environmental factors, such as meteorology.

4.2   Temporal Differences in Noise

We found that LFN does not follow the same seasonal temporal trends as A-weighted dBA loudness. At the two sites, daily average A-weighted noise metrics (LA_{eq}= A-Weighted, equivalent continuous sound level) and other time-averaged A-weighted noise descriptors (L_{DN}, L_{Night}, and L_{DEN}) were all in excess of USEPA and WHO noise thresholds (USEPA, 1974; WHO, 2009)[33,34] on all days, indicating that both sites are highly impacted by UEN (**Table1**). USEPA-recommended levels of 55 dBA (L_{DN}) were exceeded on every day of the study, as were WHO Noise Guidelines for L_{DEN} and L_{Night} (WHO, 2018) [35]. While both sites exceeded EPA and WHO guidance levels for A-weighted loudness, their frequency content and other characteristics of sound are not captured by A-weighted metrics (K.P. Waye, 2011).

Significant temporal differences in LFN were identified by two-sample t-tests, indicating that LFN dB levels are lower weekends v. weekdays, lower at night v. day, lower during non-rush hour periods v. rush hours, and lower in Spring v. Summer for the combined dataset (both sites). Sound pressure levels (SPL), measured in this study as LAeq (dBA) exhibited similar temporal characteristics. SPL and noise frequencies by site indicate that LAeq and the LFN, MFN and HFN noise frequencies are lower (dB) at Chelsea (v. Roxbury), with only VLFN dB levels higher in Chelsea v. Roxbury. At the 1-day and 1-week levels there is no difference in directionality or statistical significance for LAeq or any of the noise frequencies by site v. 30-sec averaged data.

Example spectrograms (**Fig. 2**) generated for low wind speed (<1 std below mean WS) days illustrate that the acoustic power in UEN, inclusive of transportation noise, is predominantly <160 Hz at both sites (note 60 Hz anomalies likely due to nearby 120V/240V electrical appliance interference) with VLFN dominating the soundscape in Chelsea, and Roxbury spectra showing less LFN energy on a typical, non-holiday weekend v. weekday during traffic commuting hours.

We attribute the higher VLFN levels in Chelsea to the site's transportation source mix, mainly influenced by its proximity to rail lines and close distance (2.5km) to Logan International Airport and that airport's flight path routing. Roberts (2010) attributes LFN and infrasound (VLFN) production to machinery, both rotational and reciprocating, and all forms of transport and turbulence, including pumps, compressors, [locomotive and truck] diesel engines, and aircraft [36]. Identification of LFN-emitting transportation sources utilizing tools such as machine learning is becoming a valid approach to classify source-specific temporal patterns of road traffic (e.g., peak-hour truck traffic noise)[37].

Recent work by Walker et al. (2017)[38] conducted in the Greater Boston, MA area, inclusive of this study's Roxbury site, found the highest SPL's were in the low frequency range (25 -125Hz), for n=400 samples taken at 10-minute intervals for 1 year. Additional work by Walker [39] in Chelsea in a 2021 study at n=29 sites focused on noise impacts to this EJ Community and found that Chelsea is exposed to high levels of sound, both day and night (65 dBA and 80 dBA and 90 dBA for low frequency, and infrasound sound levels sampled for 1-week durations over two seasons), with 63Hz dominant, supporting our findings.

As an example of how an extended interval length of sampling might be leveraged, we evaluated LAeq and VLFN through HFN noise frequencies for weeks when public school was in-session (school) v. not in-session (no school) in both EJC's. Our two-sample t-test results for school (n=10 weeks) v. no school (n=9 weeks) indicate that weekly-averaged loudness and noise frequencies followed seasonal trends for their respective measures by site, for data aggregated to the 1-week level. We attribute the loudness and lower frequency (VLFN and LFN) differences by site to the proximity of the site microphones to the nearest major road and differences in the local transportation mix. For example, Roxbury LAeq and VLFN (<20Hz) trends also follow seasonal trends at that site, however unlike in Chelsea, LAeq and VLFN are higher in Spring (school in session) v. Summer (school not in session) possibly due to school bus traffic along Roxbury site local roads. Conversely, Chelsea VLFN (<20Hz) is not significantly different Spring v. Summer (school v. no school), possibly due to the non-seasonal nature of Chelsea VLFN source events, e.g. aircraft, trains.

4.3   Low Frequency Noise Assessment Metrics

The literature does not universally agree upon the cutoff frequency for LFN, with values of <250Hz, <200Hz, <125Hz variously posited (E. Walker, 2017; K.P. Waye, 2002). Morsin (2018) simply groups high-frequency (>125 Hz) and low-frequency noise (<125 Hz). (Morsin, 2018, cited by Alves, 2020). European studies have modeled LFN using the LCeq-LAeq metric for road traffic noise exposure assessment and have found that a cutoff frequency of 125Hz was important when determining the percentage of exposed households (Roberts, 2010). Research by Walker et al. (2017), also in Greater Boston, utilizes the 125Hz LFN cutoff frequency. Sound below 20 Hz is generally termed infrasound (Alves, 2020) and while it may subjectively be considered a component of low-frequency noise, it is inaudible. (Bergland, 1996)[40].

To test the effect of which frequency bands LCeq-LAeq, an indicator of LFN depends on when LCeq-LAeq > 10dB (WHO,1999), we ran multivariate regression models to assess which frequency bins are contributing more significantly to LCeq-LAeq when this metric is 10dB or higher, by site. The results for 30-sec averaged data are presented in **Table 2.** For data aggregated to the 1-day level, taken together for both sites, only VLFN and LFN were significant and positive contributors to LCeq-LAeq=> 10dB (Supplementary Tables 2S and 3S, Appendix 1). Our findings support the conclusions presented by Roberts (2010), where the result of the subtraction of the two exposure levels (LCeq-LAeq) revealed the low frequency characteristic of the noise exposure, and those in a review paper by Leventhall (2003)[41] which cites the difference between C- and A-weightings (dB) is an indication of the amount of low frequency noise energy.

Our results at both the microscale (30-sec) and macroscale (1-day) data averaging levels support the use of LCeq-LAeq as an assessment tool to characterize the presence of LFN in an urban soundscape. The LCeq-LAeq metric may be more practical than spectral analysis for LFN 'screening', as LCeq values are easily gathered from sound level meters while measuring A-weighted equivalent sound pressure levels (Wang and Cray, 2013) [42]. The relative ease of obtaining these values may allow interested community residents to have a more accurate assessment of the surrounding soundscape.

4.4 Meteorological Factors Affecting Noise

In their Boston study, which sampled 400 sites in Boston (including the Roxbury site) at 15-minute intervals (February 2015- February 2016), Walker et. al (2017) found that temperature was found to be the only important meteorological predictor of increases in LFN and MFN. A Taiwanese study (Wang et. al 2016)[43] examining temporal and spatial variations in road traffic noise for different frequency components, found that average annual temperature was significantly associated with decreasing LFN road traffic noise at 31.5 Hz and 63 Hz (both p-values < 0.05). Work by Sandberg and Ejsmont (2002)[44] cites that an air temperature increase of 10°C can result in a reduction of noise emitted up to 1 dB(A).

Our study found 5 meteorological covariates (temperature, humidity, barometric pressure, wind speed and direction) were statistically significant predictors of noise outcomes of LAeq and noise frequency dB levels (VLFN, LFN, MFN and HFN), with increased humidity (%) and increased barometric pressure imparting a marginal negative effect on noise levels at both sites. Increases in temperature (deg °C) resulted in minimal positive increases in LAeq and on all noise frequency dB levels evaluated at Chelsea (LFN most effected at β = 0.252; 95% CI: 0.250, 0.254). At the 1-day and 1-week data aggregation levels, the significance and directionality of temperature on noise outcomes is unchanged for Chelsea with the exception of VLFN, on which temperature had slight negative (1-day) or insignificant (1-week) effects (Supplementary Tables 2S, 3S, Appendix 1). Temperature had insignificant or slight negative effects on Roxbury MFN and HFN dB levels, respectively, and a slight negative effect on Roxbury LAeq (β = -0.022; 95% CI: -0.023, -0.020). (**Tables 2, 3**). The Taiwanese study's (Wang et al., 2016) use of average annual temperature associations with LFN and LAeq(24-hr) v. our study's 30-s averaged temperature covariate may account for the directional differences in association with these outcomes. Aggregated to 1-day and 1-week, these directional trends and significance were similar, except temperature effects on VLFN (1-day) and LFN (1-day and 1-week) were not significant.

4.5   Assessment of Wind Effects

We found the most significant effects of high (75th percentile) wind speeds, irrespective of wind direction, were on VLFN, with a substantial increase (β = 12.5; 95% CI: 12.49, 12.58) in VLFN dB levels during high wind speeds at Chelsea; and to a lesser degree (β = 3.1; 95% CI: 3.11, 3.16) at Roxbury. LFN was minimally affected by high wind speeds at either site (**Tables 2, 3**). Conversely, in the Taiwanese study previously cited, (Wang et al. , 2016) only noise exposure at 31.5 Hz (LFN) was significantly correlated with wind speed (r=0.213; p< 0.050). We found that at the 1-day data aggregation level, wind direction and high wind speed interactions had the greatest positive effects on VLFN at both sites. At the 1-week data aggregation level no interactions of wind direction and Wind Speed HI were significant (p>0.05).

In their "Methodology for the evaluation of low-frequency environmental noise case-study," Tombolato et al., (2022) stress the importance of recording and reporting specific information regarding wind gusts, in addition to the average wind speed should become a common practice when carrying out long-term unattended (LFN) measurements [45].

## 4.6	Study Strengths and Limitations

The literature (Frank., L., et al., 2019; Glazener et al.) consistently bemoan the lack of longer-term studies, finding that most work is cross-sectional in nature. The time span of five months of ambient noise monitoring in two locations is markedly different in its depth of noise measures and meteorological measurements and available for other researchers as a .txt file possessing rich metrics, dBA, 1/3 octave - encompassing some 1 billion readings. Our rich dataset allows for aggregation levels at 30-seconds (optimized per autocorrelation algorithm) and at longer averages including 1-day and 1-week for comparison of longer intervallic trends and robust statistical tests with reduced sampling bias. Work by Ragettli et al. (2016) measuring environmental noise in Montreal affirms that bias can be reduced when sampling noise measures over a longer period (e.g. 24-hours) to effectively capture long-term average noise levels near railways and areas affected by airplane noise[46].

The use of one omni-directional sensor (microphone) at each site and therefore being unable to determine directionality of noise or perform separation of VLFN (infrasound) from wind noise is a limitation in this study, although we did perform statistical analyses of wind speed and wind direction impacts on lower frequencies to conclude that LFN presented in our study spectrograms was largely unconfounded by wind noise artifacts.

A consistent recommendation both in Glazener et al. and the overall ambient noise literature was great interest in further documenting the impact of ambient noise on "at risk" populations who are inequitably exposed. The location of the two monitoring sites (Roxbury and Chelsea – both EJ

Communities) allows for the consideration of the data through this increasingly important lens.

Only a few recent studies have evaluated community-level inequality in exposure to estimated

noise pollution. In a cross-sectional study by Casey et al., 2017 to assess racial/ethnic and socioeconomic

inequalities in noise pollution in the contiguous United States, the researchers reported a positive

association between noise levels and a community-level measure of social inequality, in this case, racial

segregation [47]. Casey et al. recommend that future work is needed to estimate how much differences in

noise exposure may explain racial disparities in noise-related health outcomes, yet the Casey study only

addresses A-weighted noise metrics as its measure of exposure. Our study thoroughly evaluates VLFN

through HFN (6.3Hz -20kHz) exposure points in two EJC's.

4.7   Summary of Key Findings

In this study we aimed to a) analyze temporal sound differences in the dataset; (b) compare and

contrast dBA noise metrics with LFN metrics in the two sites; and (c) assess meteorological covariate

contributions to LFN in the dataset. We found that LFN is predictably present as a component of UEN in

the two Environmental Justice communities studied, with statistically significant (*p-vals* <0.05) temporal

trends observed. Seasonal loudness SPL's (LAeq) varied by site, with Roxbury having higher LAeq

levels (dBA) in Spring v. Summer, and Chelsea the reverse, possibly due to disparate community noise

and differing seasonal schedules and patterns of transportation sources emitting LFN<125Hz.

We also evaluated loudness and noise frequency measures for weeks when school was in-session

v. not in-session and found similar trends to seasonality, attributing differences by site to school bus

traffic along Roxbury site local roads. The large dataset in this study is currently being tested for

implementing a machine-learning modeling approach, which will help further define spatiotemporal

differences in both loudness and noise frequencies classified by source (e.g. truck, bus, rail, aircraft).

Five meteorological covariates (temperature, humidity, barometric pressure, wind speed and

direction) were statistically significant (*p-vals* <0.05) predictors of noise outcomes of LAeq and noise

frequency dB levels (VLFN, LFN, MFN and HFN), though humidity and barometric pressure imparted slight negative effects. The most significant effect of high wind speeds, irrespective of wind direction, was on VLFN, with a substantial increase in VLFN dB levels during high wind speeds at Chelsea, and to a lesser degree at Roxbury. LFN was minimally affected by high wind speeds at either site.

5.0   Significance

5.1   Public Health Implications

Recent work by Glazener et al. (2021) synthesized information to summarize the health outcomes of transportation, along 14 identified pathways. Of interest was the prominent inclusion of ambient noise as a concern of high priority. The attributes of noise that were either directly measured or modeled skewed heavily toward sound pressure levels (SPL) or the traditional dBA set of metrics. There was little use of other attributes of noise, with no mention of LFN in the studies reviewed by Glazener et al. (2021). Alves et al. conclude in a meta-study that there are still few studies focusing exclusively on health impacts and discomfort due to LFN (Alves, et al. 2020).

Methods for measuring and quantifying LFN in the urban soundscape, while advancing technologically, are underutilized in urban noise characterization studies. With more technically advanced sound level meters (SLMs) currently available, the ability to generate spectra has greatly improved, allowing for a more whollistic view of noise frequency assessment. Visual presentation of noise spectra could be an important tool for risk communication and raising awareness of affected populations as to which temporal or diurnal periods (e.g. – rush hours) contain the highest acoustical power by frequency.

As a related example, to address the health effects of traffic noise and air pollution in nearby Somerville, MA (73% of its population reside in EJ block groups, Mass.gov, 2020), a Health Lens Analysis (HLA) was conducted, combined with a design charrette where posters and exposure maps were presented to engage affected populations near highway communities in generating proposed noise barrier approaches acceptable to the community (Brugge, D. et al., 2019) [48] .
Burger (2022) affirms in an Environmental Justice Risk Communication paper that the involvement of community members in [risk] communication is critical, especially in low-income and minority

communities, further emphasizing that there is general agreement that there are environmental risks that need to be addressed, and that need to be communicated and discussed widely (Burger, 2022) [49].

The City of Boston, MA report on the Health of Boston identifies 15 determinants that influence the health of Boston residents and communities. Of these determinants, Environmental Health is highly ranked, and includes outdoor/indoor air quality; asthma related hospitalizations; mold and asbestos violations; water leaks; second-hand smoke exposure; overcrowded housing and climate-related risks factors (heat and cold) as health-related indicators. Notably, the inclusion of dBA or LFN noise exposure is absent as a health risk determinant (City of Boston, 2016)[50]. Other major US cities have also not adequately addressed noise exposure as a public health risk. For example, *Healthy Chicago 2025*, a report which outlines a roadmap for Chicago's health and racial equity has no inclusion of UEN or noise exposure risks as threats to public health [51].

5.2   Regulatory Implications

Analysis of data presented in this study underscores the importance for urban planners and land use planners, regulatory and publc health agencies to expand their scope of mitigatating noise impacts, especially from LFN-generating sources (e.g. truck, bus, rail, aircraft). A study conducted near the present Roxbury site (Dudley Square) during 1997-2001 was used to develop a real-time State-regulatory sponsored air pollution monitoring system to test and ultimately support the hypothesis that Dudley Square in Roxbury is a hot spot for diesel-emission borne particulate air pollution. During the study dates, there were more than 15 bus and truck depots garaging more than 1,150 diesel buses and trucks within 1.5 miles of Dudley Square, as well as 25,000 people passing through its bus station daily. In addition to recommending conversion of diesel transit buses to compressed natural gas, the study bolstered the community's effectiveness in shaping local policies for transportation, development, and construction projects affecting air pollution (Pen Loh, et al, 2002) [52]. These outcomes serveas reminders of the importance of an informed citizienary in shaping environmental interventions. Burger (2022) notes that while communities at risk may experience ongoing air releases or noise, or increased traffic, risk communicators from the industry or government need to trust the community members' communications and observations of excessive exposures. Communication is key to addressing the adverse health effects, which may be able to be ameliorated, even when they cannot be immediately reduced (Burger, 2022).

Ultimately, however, LFN remains a largely unmeasured component of UEN. Not characterizing LFN and basing noise regulation on A-weightings (e.g. dBA, loudest hour) unduly exposes populations to harmful LFN levels. Therefore, the results of our study suggest that additional work be done to characterize spatiotemporal patterns of LFN in urban areas. Ultimately, this work may be such that the regulations based solely upon A-weighted noise need to be revisited.

6.0   Data Availability

The data generated and analyzed during this study are available from the corresponding author on reasonable request.

7.0   References

1. Selander, J., Bluhm, G., Theorell, T., Pershagen, G., Babisch, W., Seiffert, I., et al., 2009. Saliva cortisol and exposure to aircraft noise in six European countries.
2. Haralabidis, A.S., Dimakopoulou, K., Vigna-Taglianti, F., Giampaolo, M., Borgini, A., Dudley, M.-L., et al., 2008. Acute effects of night-time noise exposure on blood E.D. Walker et al. Environmental Research 159 (2017) 491–499 498 pressure in populations living near airports. Eur. Heart J. 29 (5), 658–664. http://dx. doi.org/10.1093/eurheartj/ehn013
3. Bodin, T., Albin, M., Ardo, J., Stroh, E., Ostergren, P.-O., & Bjork, J., 2009. Road traffic noise and hypertension: results from a cross-sectional public health survey in southern Sweden. Environ. Health 8 (1), 38–47. http://dx.doi.org/10.1186/1476- 069X-8-38.
4. Babisch, W., Beule, B., Schust, M., Kersten, N., & Ising, H., 2005. Traffic noise and risk of myocardial infarction. Epidemiology 16 (1), 33–40. http://dx.doi.org/10.1097/01. ede.0000147104.84424.24.
5. Floud, S., Vigna-Taglianti, F., Hansell, A., Blangiardo, M., Houthuijs, D., Breugelmans, O., et al., 2011. Medication use in relation to noise from aircraft and road traffic in six European countries: results of the HYENA study. Occup. Environ. Med. 68 (7),
6. Hansell, A.L., Blangiardo, M., Fortunato, L., Floud, S., de Hoogh, K., Fecht, D., et al., 2013. Aircraft noise and cardiovascular disease near Heathrow airport in London: small area study. Br. Med. J. 347. http://dx.doi.org/10.1136/bmj.f5432.
7. Correia, A.W., Peters, J.L., Levy, J.I., Melly, S., Dominici, F., 2013. Residential exposure to aircraft noise and hospital admissions for cardiovascular diseases: multi-airport retrospective study. Br. Med. J. 347, f5561. http://dx.doi.org/10.1136/bmj.f5561
8. Münzel, T., Sørensen, M., Schmidt, F., Schmidt, E., Steven, S., Kröller-Schön, S., et al., (2018). The adverse effects of environmental noise exposure on oxidative stress and cardiovascular risk. Antioxidants & redox signaling, 28(9), 873-908.
9. Münzel, T., Gori, T., Babisch, W., & Basner, M. (2014). Cardiovascular effects of environmental noise exposure. European heart journal, 35(13), 829-836.
10. Walker, E. D., Brammer, A., Cherniack, M. G., Laden, F., & Cavallari, J. M. (2016). Cardiovascular and stress responses to short-term noise exposures—A panel study in healthy males. Environmental research, 150, 391-397.
11. Waye, K. P., Clow, A., Edwards, S., Hucklebridge, F., & Rylander, R. (2003). Effects of nighttime low frequency noise on the cortisol response to awakening and subjective sleep quality. Life sciences, 72(8), 863-875.
12. Verzini, A. M., Frassoni, C. A., & Ortiz, A. H. (1999). A field study about the effects of low-frequency noise on man. The Journal of the Acoustical Society of America, 105(2_Supplement), 942-942.
13. Branco, N. A. C., Alves-Pereira, M., Araújo, A., & Reis, J. (2005). ENVIRONMENTAL VIBROACOUSTIC DISEASE–AN EXAMPLE OF ENVIRONMENTAL LOW FREQUENCY NOISE EXPOSURE. Sound and Vibration, 11, 14.
14. Araújo Alves, J., Neto Paiva, F., Torres Silva, L., & Remoaldo, P. (2020). Low-frequency noise and its main effects on human health—A review of the literature between 2016 and 2019. Applied Sciences, 10(15), 5205.
15. Ascari, E., Licitra, G., Teti, L., & Cerchiai, M. (2015). Low frequency noise impact from road traffic according to different noise prediction methods. Science of the total environment, 505, 658-669.
16. K. P. Waye, "Effects of Low Frequency Noise and Vibrations: Environmental and Occupational Perspectives," in Encyclopedia of Environmental Health, Elsevier, 2011, pp. 240–253. doi: 10.1016/B978-0-444-52272-6.00245-2
17. Glazener, A., Sanchez, K., Ramani, T., Zietsman, J., Nieuwenhuijsen, M. J., Mindell, J., et al., (2021). Fourteen pathways between urban transportation and health: A conceptual model and literature review. Journal of transport & health, 21, 101070.

18. Frank, L. D., Iroz-Elardo, N., MacLeod, K. E., & Hong, A. (2019). Pathways from built environment to health: A conceptual framework linking behavior and exposure-based impacts. Journal of Transport & Health, 12, 319-335.

19. Hasegawa, Y., & Lau, S. K. (2022). A qualitative and quantitative synthesis of the impacts of COVID-19 on soundscapes: A systematic review and meta-analysis. Science of The Total Environment, 844, 157223.

20. MASSDEP, 2020. Environmental Justice Communities in Massachusetts. Retrieved from. https://www.mass.gov/info-details/environmental-justice-communities-in-massachusetts.

21. Mass Department of Transportation (MADOT), 2016 mhd.public.ms2soft.com/tcds

22. Massachusetts Bay Transportation Authority, www.MBTA.com

23. Massachusetts Port Authority, www.massport.com

24. City of Boston, (MA), www.bostonplans.org

25. Volpe National Transportation Systems Center, US Department of Transportation, Cambridge, MA, USA PARTNER, Sleep Study #25 Acoustics System, 2014

26. General Edward Lawrence Logan International Airport (KBOS) http://www.airnav.com/airport/bos

27. Goelzer, B., cited in Hansen, C. H. (2001). Fundamentals of acoustics. Occupational Exposure to Noise: Evaluation, Prevention and Control. World Health Organization, 1(3), 23-52.

28. The Mathworks, www.mathworks.com

29. Boston University Medical Center (BUMC) IMP Amendment/Large Project Review, Howard Stein Hudson, 2013

30. Boston Public School 2016-17 District Calendar, BostonPublicSchools.org

31. WHO (1999) Guidelines for Community Noise. World Health Organization, Geneva.

32. Roberts, C. (2004, November). Ecoaccess guideline for the assessment of low frequency noise. In Proceedings of acoustics (Vol. 4).

33. US Environmental Protection Agency (USEPA), "EPA_levels_doc1978.pdf."

34. Hurtley, C. and World Health Organization, Eds., Night noise guidelines for Europe. Copenhagen, Denmark: World Health Organization Europe, 2009.

35. World Health Organization, ENVIRONMENTAL NOISE GUIDELINES for the European Region, 2018

36. Roberts, C. , "Low Frequency Noise from Transportation Sources," in Proceedings of 20th International Congress on Acoustics, 2010, pp. 23–27.

37. Wang, T., Jiang, R., Lin, Y. E., Monahan, K., Leaffer, D., Doroff, S., et al., (2021, August). Scalable Machine Learning Approach to Classifying Transportation Noise at Two Urban Sites in Greater Boston, Massachusetts. In INTER-NOISE and NOISE-CON Congress and Conference Proceedings (Vol. 263, No. 1, pp. 4962-4974). Institute of Noise Control Engineering.

38. Walker, E. D., Hart, J. E., Koutrakis, P., Cavallari, J. M., VoPham, T., Luna, M., et al., (2017). Spatial and temporal determinants of A-weighted and frequency specific sound levels—An elastic net approach. Environmental research, 159, 491-499.

39. Walker, E. D., Lee, N. F., Scammell, M. K., Feuer, A. P., Power, M. B., Lane, K. J., et al., (2021). Descriptive characterization of sound levels in an environmental justice city before and during a global pandemic. Environmental Research, 199, 111353.

40. Berglund, B., Hassmen, P., & Job, R. S. (1996). Sources and effects of low-frequency noise. The Journal of the Acoustical Society of America, 99(5), 2985-3002.

41. Leventhall, G., Pelmear, P., & Benton, S. (2003). A review of published research on low frequency noise and its effects.

42. Wang, L. M., & Kraay, B. A. (2013). Rating low levels of ambient noise in performing arts facilities.

43. Wang, V. S., Lo, E. W., Liang, C. H., Chao, K. P., Bao, B. Y., & Chang, T. Y. (2016). Temporal and spatial variations in road traffic noise for different frequency components in metropolitan Taichung, Taiwan. Environmental Pollution, 219, 174-181.

44. Sandberg, U., & Ejsmont, J.A., 2002, 'Tyre/Road Noise Reference Book'. Informex HB, Kisa, Sweden. Sa

45. Tombolato, A., Bonomini, F., & Di Bella, A. (2022). Methodology for the evaluation of low-frequency environmental noise: A case-study. Applied Acoustics, 187, 108517.

46. Ragettli, M. S., Goudreau, S., Plante, C., Fournier, M., Hatzopoulou, M., Perron, S., & Smargiassi, A. (2016). Statistical modeling of the spatial variability of environmental noise levels in Montreal, Canada, using noise measurements and land use characteristics. Journal of Exposure Science & Environmental Epidemiology, 26(6), 597-605.

47. Casey, J. A., Morello-Frosch, R., Mennitt, D. J., Fristrup, K., Ogburn, E. L., & James, P. (2017). Race/ethnicity, socioeconomic status, residential segregation, and spatial variation in noise exposure in the contiguous united states. Environmental Health Perspectives, 125(7) doi:10.1289/EHP898

48. Brugge, D., Ron, S., Reisner, E., Botana, P., Leaffer, D., Zamore, W., et al., (2019). Noise Barriers in Somerville: A Health Lens Analysis (HLA). Environmental Epidemiology, 3, 44.

49. Burger, J. (2022). Trust and consequences: Role of community science, perceptions, values, and environmental justice in risk communication. Risk Analysis, 42(11), 2362-2375.

50. Health of Boston, Snehal N. Shah, MD, MPH Director, Research and Evaluation Office, BPHC, 2016/2017 www.boston.gov

51. Healthy Chicago 2025, https://www.chicago.gov/content/dam/city/depts/cdph/statistics_and_reports/HC2025_917_FINAL.pdf

52. Loh, P., Sugerman-Brozan, J., Wiggins, S., Noiles, D., & Archibald, C. (2002). From asthma to AirBeat: community-driven monitoring of fine particles and black carbon in Roxbury, Massachusetts. Environmental Health Perspectives, 110(suppl 2), 297-301.

Chapter 4

Scalable Machine Learning Approach to Classifying Transportation Noise at Two Urban Sites in Greater Boston, Massachusetts

1. INTRODUCTION

Noise pollution in urban areas is highly associated with adverse health outcomes and deleterious effects on quality of life (Lucas de Souza and Giunta, 2011, Vlachokostas et al., 2012). Several studies have indicated that exposure to environmental noise can lead to cardiovascular risks, cognitive impairment, sleep disturbance and anxiety. (Kim et al., 2007, Belojevic et al., 1997, Belojevic et al., 2008, Hofman et al., 1995). Long term exposure to environmental noise was estimated to cause approximately 12,000 premature deaths and contribute 48,000 new cases of ischemic heart disease annually in a 32-country European study (European Environment Agency., 2020).

Transportation is one of the major sources of environmental noise, specifically sources including automobiles, airplanes, and rail (Goines and Hagler, 2007). Given increasing rates of urbanization, a larger proportion of the world's population is exposed to potentially harmful environmental noise levels which harm human health (P. De Vos, A. Van Beek, 2011). It is important to understand the temporal variability and level of exposure to transportation-associated noise as well as to the closely associated suite of air pollutants arising from the same sources.

To predict the sources of transportation-associated noise, a non-linear solution is required due to the complex multivariate relationships involved in classification and modelling (Torija & Ruiz, 2015). Machine learning (ML) methods are useful due to their non-linearity and have been effectively used to address environmental noise applications (Haykin, S, 2010).

Machine learning methods have been used extensively in noise modeling, and have been reviewed elsewhere, focusing on health impacts (Warren et al., 2006)) and urban noise mapping (Alvares-Sanches et al., (2021)). Alsouda et al. classified environmental noise data using Mel-frequency cepstral coefficients (MFCC) for audio feature extraction and supervised classification algorithms such as Support

Vector Machine (SVM) and k-Nearest Neighbors (KNN). Based on a sample size of 3000 training data inputs of sound samples grouped in eight sound classes (such as car horn, jackhammer, or street music), the peak accuracy for the SVM and KNN models ranged from 88 - 94% (Alsouda, Y., Pllana, S., et al., (2019).

Although SVM and KNN are widely utilized and result in high levels of accuracy, these traditional classifiers can only handle limited data stream variations which lack time and frequency features (Testi et al., 2018). Deep neural networks have proven to work more efficiently than conventional regression approaches. Convolutional Neural Networks (CNN) is one of the most commonly used models in environmental noise classification. CNN can successfully process voice data in structured-arrays, which address the lack of time and frequency features (Zhang et al., 2015).

Several studies have demonstrated the benefits of using CNN to classify environmental noise. Davis and Suresh (2018), Demir et al. (2020), and Mushtaq et al. (2021), obtained high accuracy and robust results that suggested CNN was extremely powerful subject to limited feature extraction and data augmentation.

The main objective of our study is to characterize transportation noise by vehicle class in two urban sites to better understand noise associations with ultra-fine particles (UFP, $<0.1\mu m$ diameter). With a better understanding of the correlation between transportation noise and UFP, particularly from diesel-fueled sources, policy makers could develop better action plans for urban structure design and minimize the joint impacts of environmental noise and air pollutants on affected populations.

2. METHODS

In this section methods of collection and pre-processing datasets are presented, to prepare the transportation-associated noise classification model. The datasets were split into individual events by finding peak values of digital samples in each audio recording.

2.1 Data collection

Tufts University (Medford, MA) researchers in Civil and Environmental Engineering (CEE), collaborated with the Volpe National Transportation Systems Center, Environmental Measurement & Modeling Division, US Department of Transportation (DOT), Cambridge, MA to plan and implement a field data collection program. The program included deployment of noise monitoring instrumentation co-located with condensation particle counters (CPC) in two Greater Boston communities impacted by vehicle and transportation-related air pollution. The monitoring sites were located at: 4 Gerrish Ave., Chelsea, MA and at the EPA Speciation Trends Network site, 1157 Harrison Ave., Roxbury, MA (Fig. 1), as a part of ongoing transportation-associated pollution studies, published elsewhere. Both sites are part of the Tufts-led Community Assessment of Freeway Exposure and Health Study (CAFEH) (Leaffer, et al., 2017).

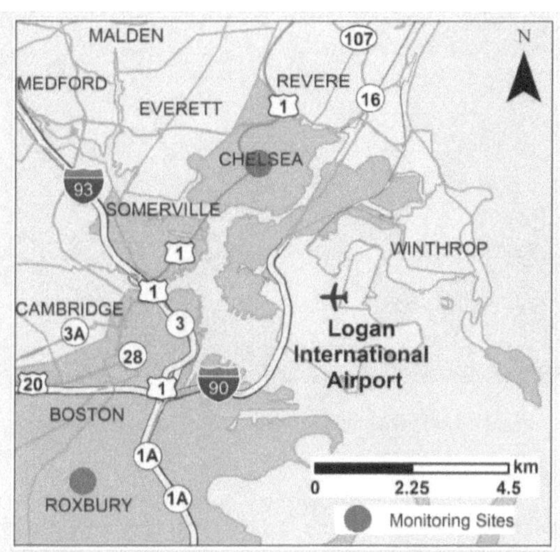

Figure 1. Map of monitoring sites (source: N.Hudda, Tufts University)

Noise monitoring was conducted with a Larson Davis 831 (LD-831) sound level meter, Larson Davis PRM831 preamplifier and a G.R.A.S. ½", free-field, pre-polarized microphone with a microphone/preamp holder. Microphones were mounted on a portable tripod and fitted with outdoor windscreens and routed with an 8-meter LD microphone cable through a Roland R-05 Digital Audio Recorder (Figure 2). Noise was sampled by the LD-831 instrument at 1 Hz resolution and stored on the LD-831 internal memory between data downloads. LD-831 data collected includes A-weighted, Z-weighted (flat) and fast time-weighted measures of sound pressure levels (SPL), maximum Z-weighted and fast time-weighted SPL and 1/3 octave band from 6.3Hz to 20kHz. Recorded, raw sound was sampled by the Roland R-05 recorder at a 44.1kHz sampling frequency and written to 32 GB SDHC cards.

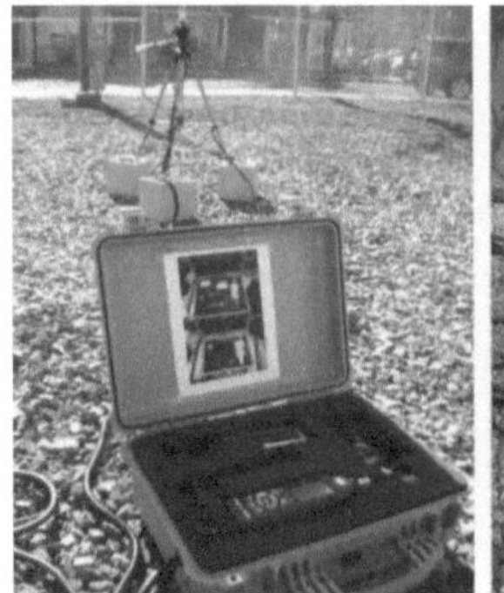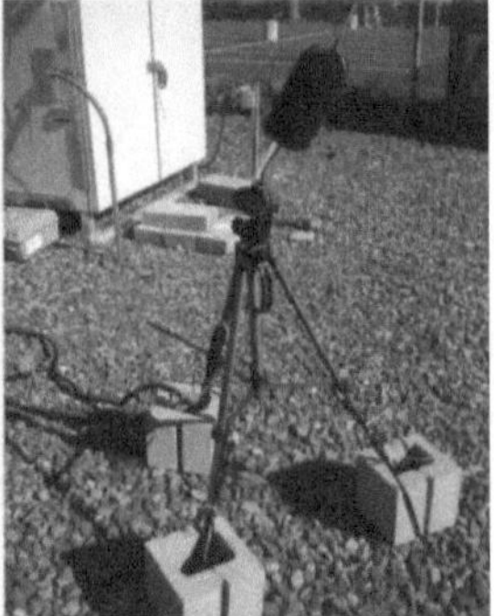

Figure 2. Microphone mounting setup (photo by author)

Given the large quantity of audio data, waveforms in the original dataset were saved as MP3 files with a high bit rate (320 kbps) to preserve as much data as possible while at the same time optimizing file size for signal processing. The collected MP3 audio files are recorded from 04/19/2016 to 09/13/2016, and the size of each file is 536.9MB. Data files were imported into MATLAB® 2021(a) engineering software ("MathWorks, Inc.," n.d.) for data visualization and analytics.

2.2 Dataset and Preprocessing

The original dataset consists of > 1850 large MP3 audio files, each with a maximum duration of 3H:43m per file. In each file, there are a wide variety of peaks associated with different noise events. Additionally, some audio files have long time sequences (e.g. – several minutes) without discernable transportation noise (Figure 3). Hence, the large audio files were split into short 'noise present' segments using an event detection algorithm in MATLAB.

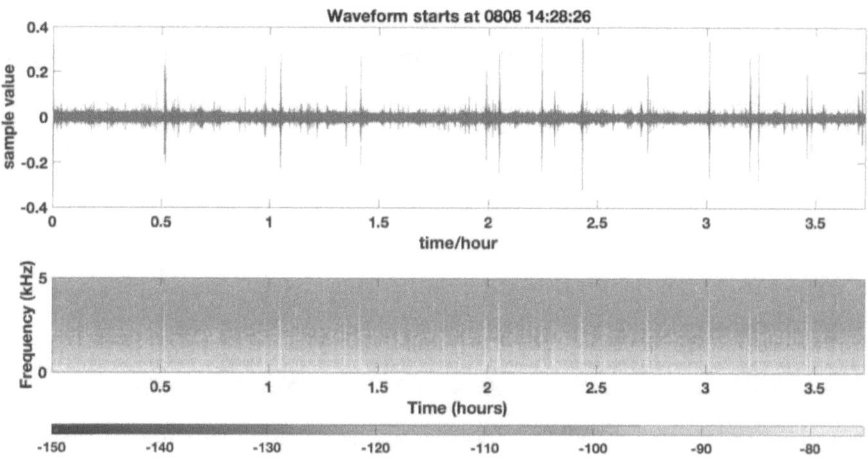

Figure 3. Example waveform and spectrogram

Each class of transportation vehicle has a variable time duration vs. peak intensity, here measured in dB, as it passes the microphone. The training files were manually split and labelled into 203 transportation sound clips or examples in the initial model. Audible confirmation of training files were validated by comparison to airport runway flight logs and local bus and rail schedules. The train-test split was 60% / 40%. We used an SGD optimizer with a learning rate of 0.01 and a momentum of 0.9. The average and maximum durations of each mode of transportation, based on n=77 events are presented in Table 1.

Table 1. Average and maximum duration for each transportation noise event

Type	Mean Duration (sec)	Standard Deviation (sec)	Maximum Duration (sec)
Truck/Bus (n=22)	7.4	8.3	24
Rail (n=45)	18.7	7.0	36
Aircraft (n=7)	12.1	14.0	35
Other (n=3)	12.0	11.1	25

Noise peaks were identified by the MATLAB function *findpeaks* in the Signal Processing Toolbox®. The code reads the raw MP3 data, acquires the upper and lower signal envelope (using the function *envelope* in the Signal Processing Toolbox), inputs the width of this envelope into *findpeaks* and returns the time index of each local peak. *MinPeakDistance* was set at 15 seconds to ignore coincident peaks.

The Short Time Fourier Transform (STFT) is one of the most frequently used noise processing and analytical tools, based on the Fourier Transform (Proakis, et al., 2001). STFT is a common-used signal processing tool that calculates by sliding an analysis window over the signal and calculate the discrete time Fourier Transform of data covered by the window. It performs well on non-random and time-varying signals in this experiment (Nawab, et al., 2001).

Spectrograms visualize frequency, time, and signal spectral characteristics, and are generated by STFT. The type of window function we selected is Hanning Window (Proakis, et al., 2001). This is a widely used window with smooth transitions and lower sidelobe, resulting in lower spectral leakage (Proakis, et al., 2001).

While creating spectrograms for machine learning training sets, the frequency axis scale should be considered, as it strongly influences the figures' spectral features. We mainly considered the linear frequency scale varying from 0-4kHz and log scale varying from 0.1-10kHz. The linear scale ranged from 0 to 4kHz since most noise energy is concentrated in this range. The log scale was selected because this scale permits visualization of low-frequency portions of the sound spectrum. For labeled images, the transport type of each image was stored in the file name of the image.

The recorded transportation events are divided into four source classifications including: rail, aircraft, truck/bus and other. Since the Chelsea site dataset (*n*=950 files) contained examples of all four source classifications, we utilized these data for model training. Example spectrograms are provided in Figure 4 (linear scale, top panel; log scale, bottom panel). The aircraft spectrograms (far left) show a clear Doppler Effect; whereas the spectral profile of the bus (middle) concentrates in the low frequency region; and the spectrum of the rail (far right) has a relatively higher power, distributed in both low- and high-frequency regions. Log scale spectrograms provided higher resolution of spectral features unique to each vehicle class.

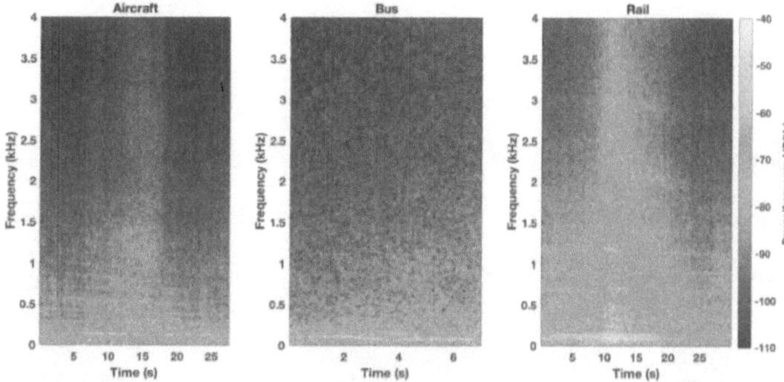

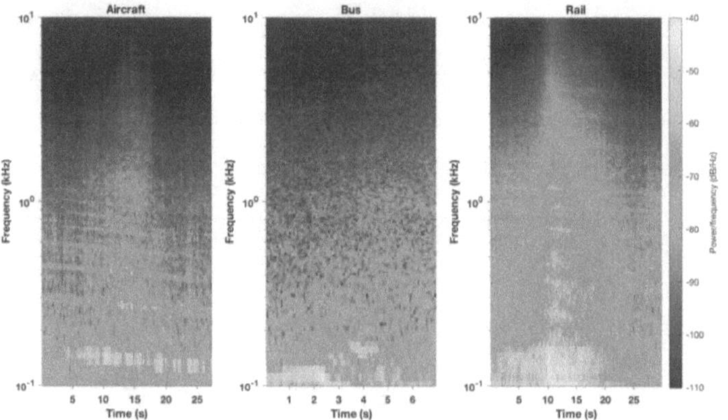

Figure 4. Example spectrograms for aircraft, bus and rail events
(linear scale, top panel; log scale, bottom panel).

2.3 Data preparation

Based on Table 1, the duration of the training data was set to be 30 seconds to effectively capture noise events, and all spectrograms were split into clips of that duration. Spectrogram images were loaded onto the High-Performance Computer cluster at Tufts University.

A selection of images from a full month of recorded sound were used, from August 8th, 2016 to September 13th, 2016, to coincide with the validation data discussed in section 2.5. These images were converted into grayscale using the *cv2* Python library and stored as *numpy* arrays with a size of 175 by 233 pixels.

2.4 Model design

All modeling training was performed using PyTorch using a NVIDIA A100 GPU and twelve cores of processing power. Two models were trained: one 4-layer CNN model, and another 125-layer *resnet34* pre-trained model. The pre-trained model had the last three layers of the CNN re-trained based on our training data. Each model was trained twice for each spectrogram scale (4k and log).

2.5 Model validation

Model validation using iterative hyperparameter selection were utilized in the model to select the momentum (0.09) and learning rate (0.01). Training validation was performed by utilizing three confirmatory sources. A first pass model training validation was conducted using field logs of visually observed transportation source pass-by events, time-stamped and logged by source (truck, train, aircraft, etc.) and peak loudness (dBA). In addition the Massachusetts Bay Transportation Authority (MBTA) commuter train timetables were consulted for validation of train arrival/departure schedules at the Chelsea site, verifying the observed v. expected time of noise events from scheduled rail transport. Lastly, the Noise Abatement Office of Logan International Airport (Massport) provided time-stamped aircraft wheels up/down flight tracking information for roughly 3000 commercial and private aircraft flights during the study period. A lag time was factored into the validation step for take-off and landing times relative to when the aircraft was detected by the Chelsea site microphone (4.0 km from airport, Figure 1). Due to the unpredictable nature of bus schedules, timetables for MBTA buses, though available for the study period, were not consulted for model validation.

3. RESULTS

Model accuracy ranges from 40.1% to 87.0% across all models (refer to Tables 2, 4). The binary classification model (Table 2) showed better results with the log scale spectrograms, with accuracy from 83.6 - 87.0%. The *resnet34* model performed better than the 4-layer CNN model, independent of spectrogram scale.

The confusion matrix for binary classification (Table 3), reports a high accuracy rate for the binary classification task (*resnet*34 model) and a majority of samples were classified correctly, with an F1 score of 0.89 (harmonic mean of the precision and recall), a measure of model quality. Confusion matrices in this study were not normalized and thus percentages do not sum to 100%.

Table 2. Binary classification (rail/no rail), accuracy %

Spectrogram scale	4-layer CNN model	125-layer *resnet*34 model
4k	50.6	51.1
log	83.6	87.0

Table 3. Confusion matrix for binary classification, accuracy %

true label		Prediction	
		rail	Other
	Rail	32.0	3.0
	Other	4.6	20.4

The multi-classification model showed similar results, with the log spectrograms producing better accuracy (65.3 - 71.0%) compared to 4k scale spectrograms (41.6 - 40.1 %) (Table 4). The 4-layer model produced slightly better results in the 4k scale, but the *resnet*34 model produced a better overall fit for the log scale.

The confusion matrix for multi-classification (Table 5) with log-scale spectrograms, *resnet*34 model showed high accuracy for rail and bus classes, but poor classification for airplane noise events.

Table 4. Multi-classification (airplane/rail/bus/truck/other), accuracy %

Spectrogram scale	4-layer CNN model	125-layer *resnet*34 model
4k	41.6	40.1
Log	65.3	71.0

Table 5. Confusion matrix for multi-classification, accuracy %

true label	Prediction				
		airplane	rail	Bus	truck	others
	airplane	1	3	2.8	0	0.4
	Rail	0	23.2	0.8	1	0
	Bus	0.2	0.8	11.4	0.8	0.8
	Truck	0	0.8	3.2	4.8	0
	Other	0.2	0	2.6	0	2.2

The last layer of the neural net is used to visualize the activation of the multiclassification CNN model, showing the areas in the spectrogram used to identify each transportation noise event (Figure 5). The saliency maps (Fig. 5 bottom panel) were produced in an effort to make the model interpretable and display where the model is focusing v. not focusing. Blue [or black] areas are where the model has low focus; red areas (high focus) display 'heat' imagery, representing an event based on model training. Pixels in red and yellow contribute to classification more saliently. Heatmaps of important regions of images aid in determining the final model predictions. This information can aid in model interpretation and can help to verify that the model is "looking" at logical predictors (e.g. engine noise, Doppler effects) of the parameters of interest (Hong, K.Y, et al., (2020).

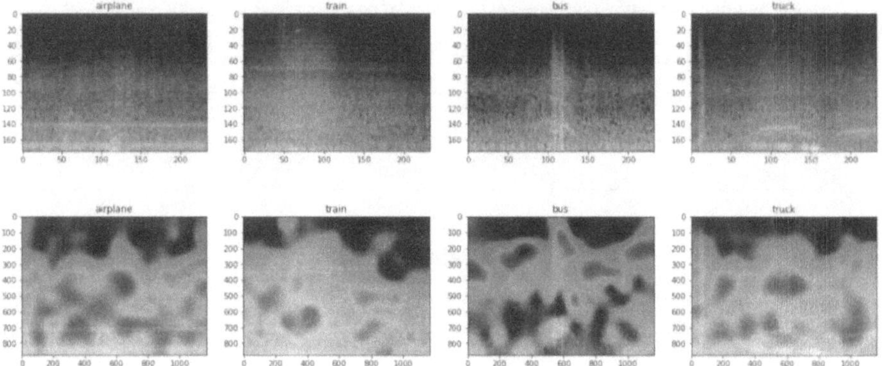

Figure 5. Heatmap of salient areas extracted from the last layer of the CNN to recognize transport noise type, each axis is in pixel units.

3.3.   Discussion

Machine learning methods have been used extensively in noise modeling, and urban noise mapping (Haykin, S, 2010, Warren et al., (2006), Alvares-Sanches et al., (2021)). The type of machine learning we utilized is intended to identify patterns of sound by source category. Our modeling approach was transfer learning, using existing models based on thousands of pieces of input data, into which we are adding spectrograms that contain Decibels, frequencies and Doppler effects for image recognition. Our model was trained on sources from their spectral features. We randomly selected 60% of our dataset to train and took the remaining 40% to test the model.

The log scale models provided a better overall fit compared to linear scale for all models tested, with the exception of the 4-layer multi-classification model which performed better at 4k scale. Saliency maps (Figure. 5), while useful to make the model interpretable and display where the model is focusing v. not focusing, were not particularly informative in this study, given the lower classification rates for images with distinctly identifiable spectral features, such as aircraft.. Given that this study team was a multi-disciplinary and multi-sectoral team (from departments including ECE, CEE, Public Health, and external consultants), saliency maps (Figure 5) can be useful for such a diverse team in understanding how the models are classifying the data and could be utilized as an aid to future work

An alternative technique to evaluate a model's efficacy at finding fragments relevant for classification via saliency maps was developed by Szczepankiewicz, K., et al. (2023). With this technique, binary ground truth (GT) masks were assigned manually or semi-automatically to each image in a diverse, specially prepared image database. The proposed indicator compares the coverage of the most relevant pixels in the saliency map with the indicated pixels in the manually prepared GT masks. However, the researchers note that while saliency maps are probably the most popular method to provide a visual explanation of decisions made by Deep Neural Network (DNN) classifiers, it is still unclear how to properly interpret saliency maps for a given image and to identify which techniques perform most accurately (Szczepankiewicz, K., et al., (2023)).

Additional work to implement cross-validation to assure validity of model results, and stratified sampling to balance the number of training data in each class, similar to work done by Poomrittigul et al. (2022) could also be considered.

In related work, our group has used the pretrained *resnet*34 model to accelerate the image-based classification and counting of specific vehicle types to be used to better understand the relationship between fine particles (PM2.5) and those vehicle types. In that study, the developed classification model was executed on a RaspberryPi 4 integrated with a Google Coral TPU coprocessor and a camera. The pre-trained (*resnet*34) model in our study performed similarly well on log spectrograms. Our work in the future will focus on a similar portable, standalone system.

Additionally, in future versions of our model we will utilize a pytorch DataLoader to set a batch size (16), with 5 epochs and a learning rate of 1E-4. We plan to utilize an adam optimizer and the *resnet*50 model, instead of the *resnet*34 model we used initially. We will run this model on A100 GPUs.

3.4 Contributions

To our knowledge, the data collected for this study is part of one of the longer duration urban environmental noise and air pollution monitoring studies to date. The modeling performed is representative of the capabilities of machine learning as applied to classifying transportation noise, potentially replacing time-consuming traffic logging done manually. Our work using sound to classify transportation sources may serve as a tool to augment video-logging of traffic. Hong, K.Y. (2020) presented a novel method of estimating spatiotemporal variations in UFP concentrations using street-level images and audio data in Montreal, Canada. Although Hong, K.Y., et al. (2020) developed models for noise as a secondary aim, the authors did not identify other studies combining street-level images and audio data to estimate outdoor air pollution concentrations.

Another strength of this study is that the sites sampled, Chelsea and Roxbury, MA, are both Environmental Justice Communities as defined by the Massachusetts Executive Office of Energy and Environmental Affairs (EEA) (mass.gov). Finally, the long temporal recordings allow for month-to-month variation in transportation noise to be accounted for in the model development.

3.5 Limitations

The limitations of our study include: 1) The models presented herein were trained to this dataset's specific noise sources and may not be generalizable to other urban areas; 2) The number of training examples (n=203) could be expanded, which would likely improve performance. Future work should include additional work on classification of airplane files to enhance the accuracy of detection of those classes; 3) although we used flight logs, MBTA schedules and visual confirmations of noise sources for confirmation of model training, we did not use these records for model validation; 4) While this study aims to inform epidemiological studies on transportation noise and associations with health, this study did not include human health data.

4. CONCLUSIONS

This study produced models of transport associated noise events with varying degrees of accuracy. Machine Learning (ML) applications presented in this study will serve to reduce dependence on the existing labor-intensive tasks such as manual playback and aural categorization of recorded sound analyzed in tandem with train schedules, traffic logs or aircraft flight schedules to synchronize and confirm sources. Additionally, these ML approaches will also reduce or eliminate human error in logging traffic counts and vehicle types.

The rich data set collected and evaluated in this study could be beneficial to development of local ordinances and policies to mitigate the dual impacts from transportation noise and air pollution on community receptors.

6. REFERENCES

1. Bravo-Moncayo, L., Lucio-Naranjo, J., Chávez, M., Pavón-García, I., & Garzón, C. (2019). A machine learning approach for traffic-noise annoyance assessment. *Applied Acoustics, 156*, 262-270.
2. de Souza, L. C. L., & Giunta, M. B. (2011). Urban indices as environmental noise indicators. Computers, Environment and Urban Systems, 35(5), 421-430.
3. Vlachokostas, C., Achillas, C., Michailidou, A. V., & Moussiopoulos, N. (2012). Measuring combined exposure to environmental pressures in urban areas: An air quality and noise pollution assessment approach. Environment international, 39(1), 8-18.
4. Kim, R. (2007). Burden of disease from environmental noise. In *WHO International Workshop on "Combined Environmental Exposure: Noise, Air Pollutants and Chemicals" Ispra.*
5. Belojević, G., Jakovljević, B., & Aleksić, O. (1997). Subjective reactions to traffic noise with regard to some personality traits. Environment International, 23(2), 221-226.
6. Belojevic, G., Jakovljevic, B., Stojanov, V., Paunovic, K., & Ilic, J. (2008). Urban road-traffic noise and blood pressure and heart rate in preschool children. Environment international, 34(2), 226-231.
7. European Environment Agency. Environmental noise in Europe, 2020. Luxembourg: Publications Office of the European Union; 2020.
8. Hofman, W. F., Kumar, A., & Tulen, J. H. M. (1995). Cardiac reactivity to traffic noise during sleep in man. Journal of sound and vibration, 179(4), 577-589.

9. Torija, A. J., Ruiz, D. P., & Ramos-Ridao, A. F. (2012). Use of back-propagation neural networks to predict both level and temporal-spectral composition of sound pressure in urban sound environments. Building and Environment, 52, 45-56.

10. Goines, L., & Hagler, L. (2007). Noise pollution: a modem plague. *South Med J*, *100*(3), 287-94.

11. Kris Y. Hong, Pedro O. Pinheiro, et al., Predicting outdoor ultrafine particle number concentrations, particle size, and noise using street-level images and audio data, Environment International, Volume 144 (2020).

12. Haykin, S. (2010). Neural networks and learning machines, 3/E. Pearson Education India.

13. Torija, A. J., & Ruiz, D. P. (2015). A general procedure to generate models for urban environmental-noise pollution using feature selection and machine learning methods. Science of The Total Environment, 505, 680–693. https://doi.org/10.1016/j.scitotenv.2014.08.060

14. Alsouda, Y., Pllana, S., & Kurti, A. (2019). IoT-based Urban Noise Identification Using Machine Learning. Proceedings of the International Conference on Omni-Layer Intelligent Systems. https://doi.org/10.1145/3312614.3312631

15. Zhang, H., McLoughlin, I., & Song, Y. (2015). Robust sound event recognition using convolutional neural networks. 2015 IEEE International Conference on Acoustics, Speech and Signal Processing (ICASSP). https://doi.org/10.1109/icassp.2015.7178031

16. Testi, E., Favarelli, E., & Giorgetti, A. (2018). Machine Learning for User Traffic Classification in Wireless Systems. 2018 26th European Signal Processing Conference (EUSIPCO). https://doi.org/10.23919/eusipco.2018.8553196

17. Zhao, M., Chang, C. H., Xie, W., Xie, Z., & Hu, J. (2020). Cloud shape classification system based on multi-channel cnn and improved fdm. IEEE Access, 8, 44111-44124.

18. Davis, N., & Suresh, K. (2018). Environmental Sound Classification Using Deep Convolutional Neural Networks and Data Augmentation. 2018 IEEE Recent Advances in Intelligent Computational Systems (RAICS). https://doi.org/10.1109/raics.2018.8635051

19. Demir, F., Turkoglu, M., Aslan, M., & Sengur, A. (2020). A new pyramidal concatenated CNN approach for environmental sound classification. Applied Acoustics, 170, 107520.

20. Mushtaq, Z., Su, S. F., & Tran, Q. V. (2021). Spectral images based environmental sound classification using CNN with meaningful data augmentation. Applied Acoustics, 172, 107581.

21. Zhao, M., Jha, A., Liu, Q., Millis, B. A., Mahadevan-Jansen, A., Lu, L., Huo, Y. (2021). Faster Mean-shift: GPU-accelerated Clustering for Cosine Embedding-based Cell Segmentation and Tracking. Medical Image Analysis, 102048.

22. Leaffer, D., Malik, R., Tracey, B., Gute, D., et. Al. (2017). Correlating transportation noise frequencies with ultrafine particulate emissions by source: Implications for environmental health studies. Proc. Mtgs. Acoust. 30, 040004 (2017); https://doi.org/10.1121/2.0000545.

23. WHO, Environmental Noise Guidelines for the European Region (2018) ISBN 9789289053563

24. Proakis, J. G. (2001). Digital signal processing: principles algorithms and applications. Pearson Education India.

25. S. Nawab, T. Quatieri and Jae Lim, "Signal reconstruction from short-time Fourier transform magnitude," in IEEE Transactions on Acoustics, Speech, and Signal Processing, vol. 31, no. 4, pp. 986-998, August 1983, doi: 10.1109/TASSP.1983.1164162.

26. Szczepankiewicz, K., Popowicz, A., Charkiewicz, K. et al., Ground truth based comparison of saliency maps algorithms. Sci Rep 13, 16887 (2023). https://doi.org/10.1038/s41598-023-42946-w26.

27. Poomrittigul, S., Chomkwah, W., Tanpatanan, T., Sakorntanant, S., & Treebupachatsakul, T. (2022, July). A comparison of deep learning CNN architecture models for classifying bacteria. In 2022 37th International technical conference on circuits/systems, computers and communications (ITC-CSCC) (pp. 290-293). IEEE.

Chapter 5

Meteorological and Spatiotemporal Associations of Urban Environmental Noise with Ultrafine Particles

1.1 • Introduction

Transportation is one of the major sources of urban environmental noise (UEN), including sources

such as automobiles, airplanes, and rail (Goines and Hagler, 2007).

Among various shared sources of air and noise pollution in an urban setting, road traffic is considered to be a main contributor to both. (EMEP/EEA, 2013). Traffic-related air pollution (TRAP) is a complex mixture of particles and gases. Exposure to TRAP is associated with increased morbidity and mortality (HEI Panel of the Health Effects of Traffic-Related Air Pollution, 2010).

Presently approximately 57% of the world's population resides in urban settlements, which are usually affected by numerous emission sources of air and noise pollution (UN, 2022). Given increasing rates of global urbanization, a larger proportion of the world's population is exposed to potentially harmful environmental noise levels, which are deleterious to human health (P. De Vos, A. Van Beek, 2011).

A recent review has shown significant associations between exposure to low-frequency noise and annoyance, sleep-related problems, concentration difficulties, and headache in the adult population living in the vicinity of noise sources (Baliatsas et al., 2016). Thus, it is important to understand the temporal variability and level of exposure to transportation-related UEN pollution as well as to the closely associated suite of TRAP emitted from the same sources (Goines, L., & Hagler, L,. 2007).

Ultrafine particles (UFPs, aerodynamic diameter <100nm), an unregulated component of TRAP, primarily derive from anthropogenic combustion sources, such as power generation and transportation activities. In urban areas, roadway traffic, rail and airport-related emissions are dominant sources of UFPs (Hudda et al., 2016), and have been the focus of exposure assessment and epidemiological studies., UFP exposure is associated with adverse cardiovascular effects including systemic inflammation biomarkers and ischemic heart disease (HEI; Boston, MA, 2013).

Since the publication of the 2010 Traffic Review (HEI, 2010) there is a better appreciation that, in addition to air pollution, many other factors are associated with traffic exposure – most notably traffic noise, and that these may either confound or modify the health effects of TRAP. Yet the questions of whether, or to what extent, the reported associations of UFP in TRAP are confounded or modified by traffic noise remain essentially uncharacterized.

1.2   Background

In one of the first investigations of the relationship between traffic-related air pollution and noise in the US, Allen, et al., (2009) found that wind direction was an important modifier of the relationships between air pollution (UFP, NO, NO_2) and noise (5-min A-weighted equivalent continuous sound pressure levels ($LAeq_{(5-min)}$)), also concluding that noise was minimally impacted by wind direction at two urban sites in Chicago, IL and Riverside, CA. Ross, Z., et al., (2011) found that noise levels at a high-traffic urban site in NYC are temporally correlated with traffic and elemental carbon and correlations are modified by the time of day, noise frequency and wind.

Despite extensive study of the effects of spatiotemporal factors on variation in transportation noise, links between transportation noise and UFP have not been well defined. In a study by Can, Rademaker et al., predictive models were developed to estimate UFP (measured as total particle number) adjusted for meteorological conditions for specific noise indicators ((L_{125Hz}- L_{2KHz}) = low to medium frequency noise bands). These models showed strong correlation (Spearman's r=0.62) between measured and predicted TPN based on wind speed and wind direction. A key constraint in the development and refinement of such models is the difficulty in measuring noise frequencies that are fully representative of traffic sources, rather than reliance on the conventional A-weighted (dBA) sound pressure levels (SPL) for model construction (Can, A., Rademaker et al., 2011).

In their review of road traffic noise exposure assessment, Khan, J. et al., (2018) conclude from a selection of 57 articles of 858 screened that air and noise pollution propagate very differently spatiotemporally and they are not necessarily highly correlated. Therefore, they should be modelled separately and cannot serve as proxy for each other. As a qualifier to this conclusion, these 57 studies (four of which assessed UFP) all utilized A-weighted (dBA) noise metrics.

Dekoninck et al., (2016) affirm that the correlation between noise and particulate matter exposure is complex yet could be improved. For example, Dekoninck et al. note that noise measurements contain spectral information that is highly relevant to improve this correlation, and specific noise indicators could be derived for this purpose. Dekoninck et al. add that simultaneous noise and black carbon (BC) and UFP measurements add significant value to predictions of air pollution models (Dekoninck, et al., 2016).

Models linking UEN frequencies, rather than dBA, to emissions of UFP components of TRAP may hold promise to help disentangle the independent health effects of the two pollutants in epidemiological studies.

1.3   Objectives

To better understand the relationships between UFP concentrations, transportation-related noise frequencies, and meteorology in urban neighborhoods we have undertaken an investigation of the associations of UEN loudness and frequencies with particle number concentration (PNC, a proxy for UFP). In this study we measured sound pressure levels (SPL), noise emission spectra, PNC, and meteorology continuously for five months in two urban sites in metropolitan Boston (Massachusetts, USA).

Our objectives were to (1) establish whether loudness and noise frequencies emitted from urban noise sources identified by metrics such as 1/3-octave band spectral analysis are associated with PNC, controlling for meteorology, time of day and site; and to (2) determine if effect modification of the noise-PNC association is moderated by impact sector wind parameters (i.e., from the direction of transportation noise – airport, roadways, rail lines, bus station) has statistically significant associations with elevated *ln*(PNC) compared to non-impact sector winds; and 3) to develop a model of PNC outcomes with predictive covariates of noise and noise frequencies and their interaction with wind parameters, and 4) to support validation of this model from studies by others at the two sites which also measured PNC and meteorology.

2.0   Materials and Methods

2.1   Study Areas

We measured noise and PNC at two urban sites between April 15 and September 13, 2016. Both sites are located in Environmental Justice Communities (EJC) burdened with multiple environmental stressors (e.g., close proximity to major road, rail and air networks) (Walker, et al., 2021).

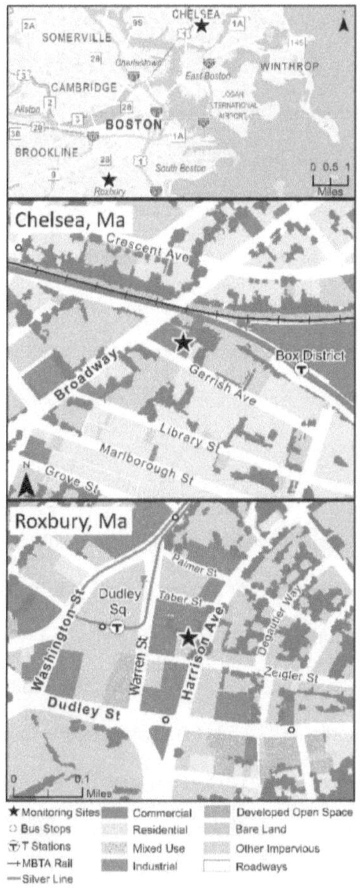

Fig. 1 Location of Noise Monitoring Sites

Monitoring sites are shown as black star symbols. Land use categories are illustrated by zoning type or physical features. Locations of bus stops, bus routes and rail (MBTA, T Stations) are indicated by icons. The lower two panels share the same scale bar.

One site was in Chelsea, a city north of Boston (**Figure 1**). Chelsea has a population of 40,615

and a population density of 7,096/km^2, making it the second most densely populated city in

Massachusetts (census, 2020). The City of Chelsea is intersected by a major expressway (U.S. Route 1),

bus and commuter rail lines, and aircraft flight paths departing and arriving at Logan International Airport

(**Fig. 1**). Noise and PNC monitoring instrumentation at the Chelsea site were located atop of a 3-story

building (10 m. above grade) located 45 m from a busy street (approx. 7300 total vehicles/day

(VPD)(Mass DOT, 2016), 50 m from rail lines (67 trips/day (TPD) (mbta.com, *2016*) and 4.0 km (NW)

from Logan International Airport (1100 flights/day in study year 2016) (Massport.com, 2016).

The second site was at the USEPA Chemical Speciation Monitoring Station (EPA site code#

250250042) in Roxbury (**Figure 1**). Roxbury is a neighborhood of Boston with a population of 51,252

(City of Boston, 2015) and a population density of 5,344/km^2. The Roxbury noise and PNC monitoring

site is located at street level, 15 m from a commercial/residential roadway (approx. 8000 total VPD, City

of Boston, 2015), 7.3 km (SW) from Logan Airport and 75 m from a city bus terminal (~250 buses/day

(mbta.com)).

2.3   Measurement Methods

Noise monitoring was conducted using two identical Larson Davis 831 (LD-831) Class 1 sound

meters, each equipped with a preamplifier (LD-PRM831) and a G.R.A.S. 1-cm free-field, pre-polarized

microphone. Microphones were mounted on 1.5-m-high tripods fitted with outdoor windscreens and

routed with 8-m microphone cables through a Roland R-05 Digital Audio Recorders. Raw sound was

recorded by the Roland R-05 recorder at a 44.1 kHz sampling frequency and written to 32 GB SDHC

cards. Given the large quantity of audio data (>1850 raw sound files), waveforms were saved as .mp3

files with a high bit rate (320 kbps) to preserve as much data as possible while at the same time managing

file size.

The Chelsea microphone was oriented upwards, perpendicular to its roof-mounted installation

surface; the Roxbury microphone was oriented due south, towards Harrison Avenue, at a 45-degree angle

to the horizontal. The sound meters measured sound pressure levels in decibels (dB) continuously over a

frequency range of 6.3 Hz to 20 kHz at 1-second (s) intervals.

Co-located with the noise monitoring instruments at each site were condensation particle counters

(CPCs, model 3783, TSI; 7-3000nm) to measure PNC and Davis VantagePro weather stations, which recorded wind speed, wind direction, temperature, relative humidity, barometric pressure, and rainfall. The CPC recorded 30-second PNC readings.

2.3 Quality Assurance

Quality assurance (QA) methods were adapted from the Protocol for a Sleep Study (PARTNER, #25, 2014). Prior to deployment, the sound meter was field-calibrated with a B&K 4231 sound level calibrator and microphone simulator to 94 dB and 114 dB at 1 Hz. Weekly calibration checks were conducted at both sites under the same protocol. Measurements were stored on the internal memory of the sound meters and downloaded weekly. Instrument clocks were set against the National Institute of Standards and Technology (NIST) atomic clock; clock drift was +/-0.75 s/day for the sound meters and +1.4 to +2.9 s/day for this digital audio recorders. Clock drift adjustments were addressed in the resampling of the raw noise data to synchronize with the CPC and meteorological data.

Weekly field checks of the meteorology station included data downloads, battery power logs and clock resets to NIST time. CPCs were calibrated annually at TSI, and side-by-side tests conducted in our laboratory for related studies of PNC in the Boston area indicate a good agreement ($r^2 = 0.97$) (Hudda et al., 2016). CPC time clocks drifted < 1 min/week to NIST time. Weekly field checks of the on-site (Davis VantagePro) meteorology stations included data downloads and battery power logs. Meteorological data were checked for comparability against Logan Airport, Boston historical weather records (FAA Identifier KBOS).

2.4 Data Processing

Noise measures evaluated in this study included A-weighted ($LAeq_{(time)}$, dB(A)) and unweighted (or Z-weighted, independent of frequency) 1/3-octave band readings collected from 6.3 Hz – 20 kHz, continuously at 1-s intervals. (Goelzer et al., 2001). Average binned levels for infrasound, or very low frequency noise (VLFN<20 Hz); low frequency noise (LFN, 20 – 125 Hz), medium frequency noise (MFN, 125 – 500 Hz), and high frequency noise (HFN >500Hz) were calculated as presented in a previous study (Leaffer et al., 2023).

PNC data were reviewed for very low concentrations (<500 particles/cm3) and measurements automatically flagged by the instrument (e.g., due to nozzle clogs and low pulse heights), per protocols established at our laboratory by Simon et al., (2017). Data marked with these flags and/or pulse heights <800 mV were removed (<1 std below mean instrument pulse height)(Simon, M., 2017).

Raw 1-s noise LAeq(time) data were aggregated to 1-min averages for the statistical analysis per an autocorrelation algorithm designed to reduce correlations between successive 1-s samples in a vector by 50% with a 60-sec lag time (VLFN and LFN were decorrelated to >33% at the 60-sec time averaging interval). Autocorrelation lag-time plots are found in the Supplementary Materials of this paper (Appendix 2). Research by Boogard et al., 2009 on exposure to ultrafine and fine particles and noise during cycling and driving in 11 Dutch cities aggregated all data covariates to 1-minute averages, noting that correlations between PNC and noise were moderate (0.21–0.60) when 1-minute averages were compared (Boogard et al., 2009).

Chelsea and Roxbury noise, meteorology and PNC measurements were all resampled to 1-min averages. Work by Simon et al., (2017) in the same geographies as our study (Chelsea, Roxbury) also aggregated PNC data to 1-min averages, noting that at longer averaging periods, the effects of transient PNC spikes from local sources (e.g., vehicles) were smoothed out (Simon, M., et al., 2017). Ragettli (2016) cites strong correlations (r=0.85) between 5-minute and 24-hour road traffic noise (LAeq(24-hr)) and moderate correlations (r=0.56 to r=0.6) for rail and air, suggesting that the continuous nature of road traffic noise is suitable for shorter duration (5-minute) sampling. Ragettli additionally notes that 2-minute noise sampling intervals may present limitations in capturing discontinuous noise events from trains and aircraft (Ragettli, M., et al., (2016)). We selected 1-minute sampling averages in our study to minimize such limitations.

Spearman correlation tables of noise and meteorology covariates at 1-min intervals for Logan Airport (KBOS) weather data are presented in **Table 1** and by site in **Table 2**.

Table 1   **Noise and Meteorological Data Correlations**

Logan Airport Meteorology Dataset (n=106,103 rows)

Covariate	LAeq$_{(1-min)}$	VLFN	LFN	MFN	HFN	Temp	Humidity	Wind Speed
LAeq$_{(1-min)}$	--	0.260	0.750	0.890	0.987	0.077	-0.049	0.104
VLFN	0.260	--	0.470	0.354	0.253	0.083	-0.264	0.501
LFN	0.750	0.470	--	0.803	0.703	0.218	-0.167	0.227
MFN	0.890	0.354	0.803	--	0.849	0.144	-0.101	0.152
HFN	0.987	0.253	0.703	0.849	--	0.082	-0.020	0.096
Temp°C	0.077	0.083	0.218	0.144	0.082	--	-0.133	0.103
Humidity%	-0.049	-0.264	-0.167	-0.101	-0.020	-0.133	--	-0.264
Wind Speed (kmph)	0.104	0.501	0.227	0.152	0.096	0.103	-0.264	--

Note: p-vals all <0.05
LAeq$_{(1-min)}$ = A-weighted sound pressure levels (dBA); Very Low Frequency Noise, VLFN(<20Hz); Low Frequency Noise, LFN(20-125Hz); Medium Frequency Noise, MFN(125-500Hz); High Frequency Noise, HFN(>500Hz)

Table 2   **Noise and Meteorological Data Correlations by Site**

Chelsea site   *Logan Airport Meteorology Dataset (n=40,770 rows)*

Covariate	LAeq$_{(1-min)}$	VLFN	LFN	MFN	HFN	Temp	Humidity	Wind Speed
LAeq$_{(1-min)}$	--	0.417	0.780	0.914	0.987	0.463	-0.043	0.237
VLFN	0.417	--	0.519	0.428	0.398	0.109	-0.203	0.648
LFN	0.780	0.519	--	0.797	0.742	0.454	-0.094	0.341
MFN	0.914	0.428	0.797	--	0.858	0.443	-0.123	0.248
HFN	0.987	0.398	0.742	0.858	--	0.487	-0.026	0.228
Temp°C	0.463	0.109	0.454	0.443	0.487	--	-0.111	0.084
Humidity%	-0.043	-0.203	-0.094	-0.123	-0.026	-0.111	--	-0.220

Wind Speed (kmph)	0.237	0.648	0.341	0.248	0.228	0.084	-0.220	--

Note: *p-vals all <0.05 for correlation coefficients*

Roxbury site   *Logan Airport Meteorology Dataset (n=40,770 rows)*

Covariate	LAeq$_{(1\text{-}min)}$	VLFN	LFN	MFN	HFN	Temp	Humidity	Wind Speed
LAeq$_{(1\text{-}min)}$	--	0.458	0.551	0.815	0.976	-0.239	-0.131	0.076
VLFN	0.458	--	0.721	0.606	0.411	0.060	-0.312	0.400
LFN	0.551	0.721	--	0.720	0.461	0.093	-0.294	0.218
MFN	0.815	0.606	0.720	--	0.751	-0.103	-0.178	0.158
HFN	0.976	0.411	0.461	0.751	--	-0.249	-0.067	0.054
Temp°C	-0.239	0.060	0.093	-0.103	-0.249	--	-0.160	0.116
Humidity%	-0.131	-0.312	-0.294	-0.178	-0.067	-0.160	--	-0.292
Wind Speed (kmph)	0.076	0.400	0.218	0.158	0.054	0.116	-0.292	--

Note: *p-vals all <0.05 for correlation coefficients*

3.0   Model Building

3.1   Statistical Analyses

Simple and multivariate regression models were run in MATLAB for noise, PNC and meteorological covariates resampled to 1-min, using Logan Airport (KBOS) weather data given generally lower covariate correlation values v. on-site meteorological parameters (**Table 1**). Covariates with Spearman's rho coefficients $r>0.65$ – indicating a high degree of correlation (**Tables 1, 2**) - were not included in the regression models due to collinearity. Summary statistics for covariates selected for simple and multivariate regression models are tabulated in **Table 3**.

Table 3   **Noise, PNC and Meteorological Data Summary Statistics**

Chelsea site (n=151 days)

Noise Covariate	Unit	Minimum	5th Pctl	Mean	STD	Median	95th Pctl	Maximum

$LA_{(eq)(1\text{-}min)}$	dB(A)	44.0	49.1	55.4	3.7	55.3	61.4	75.7
VLFN (<20 Hz)	dB	48.0	53.9	65.6	8.5	64.1	81.7	99.1
LFN (20 125 Hz)	dB	56.7	62.1	67.9	3.8	68.0	74.0	90.1
MFN (125-500 Hz)	dB	47.8	51.7	57.1	3.5	56.9	62.9	78.1
HFN (>500 Hz)	dB	48.3	50.4	54.9	3.0	54.5	60.0	76.0
PNC	# particles/cc	1845	2620	9650	5777	8225	21550	27850

Roxbury site (n=151 days)

Noise Covariate	Unit	Minimum	5th Pctl	Mean	STD	Median	95% Pctl	Maximum
$LA_{(eq)(1\text{-}min)}$	dB(A)	52.1	56.5	60.1	2.3	60.0	63.7	83.4
VLFN (<20 Hz)	dB	51.2	55.7	63.1	4.1	63.4	69.5	93.0
LFN (20 -125 Hz)	dB	61.4	66.2	71.9	3.1	72.3	76.4	88.6
MFN (125 -500 Hz)	dB	54.6	57.5	60.3	2.0	60.1	63.9	79.9
HFN (>500 Hz)	dB	50.2	55.2	58.7	2.3	58.6	62.3	83.1
PNC	# particles/cc	1355	5466	19688	12997	16550	44250	159000

Meteorology*

Covariate	Unit	Minimum	5th Pctl	Mean	STD	Median	95th Pctl	Maximum
Wind Speed	km/hr	0	0	15.2	7.5	14.8	29.6	42.6
Temperature	deg °C	2.8	6.7	16.3	7.5	16.1	28.3	36.1
Humidity	%	12.7	31.1	61.7	19.5	60.8	92.8	100
Visibility	km	0.39	9.6	15.4	2.5	16.0	16.1	16.1

Notes: *LAeq(time)* = A-weighted, equivalent continuous sound level (time period), VLFN (<20Hz), LFN (20 -125Hz), MFN (125Hz -500Hz), HFN (>500Hz), PNC (outliers removed) and meteorological parameters resampled to 1-min.
*Meteorological data from (KBOS) Logan International Airport.

3.2   Regression Covariate Selection

Base models were run for each of the five noise measures together with key covariates (e.g. temporal factors, site, and meteorological parameters). Meteorological variables considered for the base models included temperature (°C), humidity (%) and wind speed (km/hr). Visibility (km) was used for a correlation analysis with PNC. Wind direction was used in multivariate regression models to classify data as impact or non-impact sector. Patton et al. (2015) found that wind direction sectors that included the airport as an upwind source were a significant explanatory variable for PNC in communities located 4–8 km north-northwest (NNW) of Logan airport (Patton et al., 2015). Temporal covariates included in the models were time of day (day==0700-2300 hrs; night==2300-0700 hrs). The Supplementary Materials of this paper include a summary of all models run (Appendix 2).

3.3   Regression Model Building

Multivariate regression models were run in MATLAB R.2023a (Mathworks.com). PNC measures were natural log-transformed *ln*(PNC) to mitigate the impact of outliers (Simon et al., 2017) and per PNC regression model building criterion reported by Patton et al., (2015) which also log-transformed PNC data (Patton, A. et al., 2015).

Work by Dekoninck et al. (2013) developing an instantaneous spatiotemporal model to predict a bicyclist's Black Carbon (BC) exposure based on mobile noise measurements used a logarithm of BC as an outcome variable since noise is also measured on a logarithmic scale (Dekoninck, et al., 2013).

Models were run to (1) establish whether loudness and noise frequencies emitted from urban noise sources identified by metrics such as 1/3-octave band spectral analysis are associated with statistically significant variations in *ln*(PNC), controlling for meteorology, time of day and site; and to (2) determine if effect modification of the noise-PNC association moderated by impact sector wind parameters (i.e. from direction and sources of transportation noise – airport, roadways, rail lines, bus station) has statistically significant associations with elevated *ln*(PNC) compared to non-impact sector winds.

4.0   Results and Discussion

4.1   Summary of Regression Model Results

Regression model results (**Table 3**) indicate that a model comprised of lower noise-frequencies (VLFN, LFN) and their interactions with wind speed performed better (AIC: 9.6E3; R^2= 0.27) at predicting *ln*(PNC) than a dBA-only model with LAeq($_{1-min}$) and a dBA:wind speed interaction model (AIC: 1.03E4; R^2=0.16). Models were controlled for wind impact sector from Logan Airport, a known source of elevated PNC emissions (Patton et al., 2014, 2015; Hudda et al., 2016; Simon, et al., 2017).

Similar results were found for models predicting *ln*(PNC) with wind impact sectors from local roadways. Lower noise-frequency (VLFN, LFN) models and their interactions with wind speed also performed better (AIC: 1.77E4; R^2= 0.22) at predicting *ln*(PNC) than a dBA-only model (AIC: 1.87E4; R^2= 0.15). Additional models of C-weighted (nearly independent of frequency) minus A-weighted decibels, LCeq-LAeq($_{24-hr}$) when paired with dBA and wind speed were not significant predictors (p>0.05) of *ln*(PNC).

Generally, VLFN imparts slight negative effects on *ln*(PNC), depending on wind speed and impact sector wind direction (airport, roadways, rail lines, bus station), while LFN imparts positive effects of a similar magnitude. In models with either VLFN or LFN, overall sound pressure levels, measured as LAeq($_{1-min}$) (dBA) have positive effects on *ln*(PNC).

Impact sector winds were important determinants of *ln*(PNC), with the strongest positive effects from winds from the direction of Logan Airport and from the railway at the Chelsea site for noise measures modeled. In Roxbury, the interaction effects of impact sector winds from Harrison Ave. (**Figure 1**) and from the Nubian Square MBTA (T) bus station had significant positive associations with *ln*(PNC) for VLFN (road) and LFN and LAeq($_{1-min}$) (bus station). Other meteorological covariates - temperature, humidity (%) and wind speed - were modeled, but only wind speed==HI (75th percentile) strongly affected model results for various noise covariate associations with *ln*(PNC).

Site and site interactions with noise measures and time of day were also significant predictors of ln(PNC), with time of day (Day==1, or 0700-2300HRS) effect estimates nearly unchanged in every model run. **Table 5S** (Supplementary Materials, Appendix 2) present the results of our regression models evaluating effect modification by noise covariates, temporal factors and meteorological factors on ln(PNC).

Table 4   **Wind Robust Multivariate Regression Model Coefficients**

Model	Covariates	Effect Est.	Adj. R^2	*p-val*	AIC
*1. ln(PNC) ~ β₀ + β₁*LAeq(1-min) + e*	Intercept	5.66	0.158	0	1.03+04
Impact Wind from Airport (n=5000 obs.)	LAeq(1-min)	0.07		<0.001	
*Predicted PNC = 18,946 #/cm^3					
*2. ln(PNC) ~β₀ +β₁*LAeq (1-min) +LAeq:WS+ e*	Intercept	5.46	0.162	<0.001	1.03+04
Impact Wind from Airport (n=5000 obs.)	LAeq(1-min)	0.07		<0.001	
	LAeq:WS	-0.0001		<0.001	
*Predicted PNC = 19,252 #/cm^3					
*3. ln(PNC) ~β₀ +β₁*LAeq (1-min) +VLFN + e*	Intercept	5.72	0.157	<0.001	1.04+04
Impact Wind from Airport (n=5000 obs.)	LAeq(1-min)	0.072		<0.001	
	VLFN	-0.0021		0.32	
*Predicted PNC = 21,692 #/cm^3					
4. ln(PNC) ~β₀ +β₁+VLFN + LFN*WS + e*	Intercept	3.29	0.273	<0.001	9.61+03
Impact Wind from Airport (n=5000 obs.)	VLFN	-0.027		<0.001	
	LFN	0.0119		<0.001	
	LFN:WS	-0.0001		<0.001	
*Predicted PNC = 19,270 #/cm^3					
*5. ln(PNC) ~ β₀ + β₁*LAeq(1-min) + e*	Intercept	6.32	0.148	0	1.87+04
Impact Wind from Roadway (n=11,515 obs.)	LAeq(1-min)	0.056		0	
*Predicted PNC = 14,496 #/cm^3					
*6. ln(PNC) ~β₀ +β₁*LAeq (1-min) +LAeq:WS+ e*	Intercept	5.45	0.162	<0.001	1.03+04
Impact Wind from Roadway (n=11,515 obs.)	LAeq(1-min)	0.077		<0.001	
	LAeq:WS	-0.00013		<0.001	
*Predicted PNC = 20,268 #/cm^3					
*7. ln(PNC) ~β₀ +β₁*LAeq (1-min) +VLFN + e*	Intercept	6.86	0.164	0	1.86+04
Impact Wind from Roadway (n=11,515 obs.)	LAeq(1-min)	0.061		0	
	VLFN	-0.0125		<0.001	
*Predicted PNC = 32,665 #/cm^3					

Note: *Models 1-4 utilize median values: LAeq(1-min)=58.8dBA; VLFN=62.7dB; LFN=70.6dB; wind speed (WS)=13.0km/hr;*
Models 5-8 utilize median values: LAeq(1-min)=58.2dBA; VLFN=64.2dB; LFN=70.6dB; wind speed (WS)=16.7km/hr

4.2 Noise Covariate, Meteorological and Spatiotemporal Effects on *ln*(PNC)

Regression models (Supplementary **Table 5S**, Models 1-6, Appendix 2) were run to establish whether loudness and noise frequencies emitted from urban noise sources identified by metrics such as 1/3-octave band spectral analysis are associated with PNC concentrations, including meteorological and temporal covariates and site interactions with noise.

Comparing noise covariate models run for VLFN and LAeq($_{1\text{-min}}$) (Model 1) and VLFN and LFN (Model 2), and adding temperature, humidity (%) and time of day (Day==1 is 0700-2300HRS) we found that VLFN had a negative association with *ln*(PNC) in both models, while LFN and LAeq($_{1\text{-min}}$) had positive associations. Both temperature ($^{\circ}$C) and relative humidity (%) had slight negative associations with *ln*(PNC) in these models. Site (Roxbury==1) had strong negative effects on *ln*(PNC) v. Chelsea, while interactions of site and VLFN, LFN and LAeq($_{1\text{-min}}$) all had slight positive effects. Model 2 had a lower AIC value and higher R^2 vs. Model 1 (see **Table 5**), implying models with lower frequencies of noise (VLFN and LFN) as covariates should have improved prediction of *ln*(PNC) vs. models with loudness as a covariate.

We also investigated correlations between PNC and visibility. Spearman's rho correlations for visibility (km) and PNC (#/cc) were r=0.19 for Chelsea; r=0.04 for Roxbury. Controlled for wind speed (WS_HI = 75th percentile) these correlations were r=0.06 for Chelsea WS_HI, r = 0.29 for Chelsea controlled for stagnant winds. Spearman's rho correlations for Roxbury, controlling for wind speeds were r= 0.03 for Roxbury WS_HI), and r = 0.10 controlled for stagnant winds. Stagnant winds were defined by Young et. al. (2023) as <1.1 m/s in a study of visibility impacts of ambient sub-micrometer particle number size distributions in an urban area of central Taiwan (Young, i-Hao, et. al. (2023)).

4.3 Effects of Noise and Wind Speed and Wind Direction on *ln*(PNC)

In Models 3 through 6 (**Table 5S**, Supplementary Materials, Appendix 2) we evaluated effects of VLFN, LFN and LAeq($_{1\text{-min}}$) on *ln*(PNC), controlling for wind speed. Effect modifications of wind speed==LO (upper quartile) in Models 3 and 5 differed little in their magnitude and direction of effect estimates and significance from base Models 1 and 2 not controlling for wind speed. The exception to this was the interaction of LAeq:site in wind effect modifications Model 3 (β = -0.007, 95% ci (-0.010, -0.004), $p<0.001$) vs. Model 1 (β = 0.028, 95% ci (0.024, 0.030), $p<0.001$), where the Model 1 effect estimate β coefficient increased 5-fold in the positive direction from Model 3 under controlled wind speed conditions. Model 3 also had a lower AIC value and higher R^2 vs. Model 1, here implying the model controlling for wind speed==LO should have improved prediction of *ln*(PNC) vs. models not controlling for wind speed.

Comparing effect modification models (Models 4 and 6) for wind speed==HI (75th percentile), we found significant differences in effect estimates vs. base Models 1 and 2 not controlling for wind speed. The more important of these differences are the effect estimate of low frequency noise (LFN 20-125 Hz) in Model 6 was not significant (β = 0.002, 95% ci (-0.002, 0.006), $p=0.28$), nor were the interaction effects of VLFN:site (β= -0.0004 95% ci (-0.003, 0.002), $p=0.80$) under wind speed==HI conditions. We also found that the temperature (°C) effect estimate increased in magnitude 125% in the positive direction from Model 3 (β = -0.008, 95% ci (-0.009, -0.007), $p<0.001$) to Model 4 (β = 0.002, 95% ci (0.0012, 0.003), $p<0.001$) as wind speeds increased from LO (upper quartile) to HI (75th percentile) for models including LAeq($_{1\text{-min}}$) and VLFN with site, time of day and humidity (%).

4.3.1   Effect Modifications of Wind Direction on *ln*(PNC)

Models 7 through 10 (**Table 5S**, Supplementary Materials, Appendix 2) were run to assess the effect modifications of impact wind effects on *ln*(PNC) outcomes by site. We defined wind impact sectors in our study as those previously presented by Hudda et al. for the same study areas (Hudda et. al., 2016).

4.3.1.1 Effect Modifications of Wind Direction from Logan Airport

For the Chelsea site, we found that during impact sector winds from Logan Airport (wind direction SE: 135 -175°), both $LAeq_{(1-min)}$ and LFN had positive interaction effect estimates with wind direction on ln(PNC) in models also including Day==1 (0700-2300HRS) as a covariate (Model 7, LAeq:Wind_Impact_Logan: $\beta = 0.013$, 95% ci (0.007, 0.018), $p<0.001$); (Model 8, LFN:Wind_Impact_Logan: $\beta = 0.020$, 95% ci (0.015, 0.025), $p<0.001$).

At the Roxbury site, we found that the effect estimate for VLFN when the wind impact sector was from Logan Airport (Model 9) was not significant ($\beta = -0.006$, 95% ci (-0.01, 0.01), $p=0.056$). In Model 10 assessing effect modifications of impact sector winds in Roxbury, LFN alone was not significant ($\beta = -0.0005$, 95% ci (-0.003, 0.002), $p=0.693$), yet the interaction of LFN:Wind_Impact_Logan was significant in this model ($\beta = 0.013$, 95% ci (0.005, 0.02), $p<0.001$).

4.3.1.2 Effect Modifications of Wind Direction from Railway

Models of impact sector winds from the railway, located north of the Chelsea site showed that only VLFN had positive interaction effect estimates with wind direction on ln(PNC) in models also including Day==1 (0700-2300HRS) and $LAeq_{(1-min)}$ or LFN, respectively as covariates (Model 7, VLFN:Wind_Impact_Rail: $\beta = 0.019$, 95% ci (0.017, 0.021), $p<0.001$); (Model 8, VLFN:Wind_Impact_Rail: $\beta = 0.022$, 95% ci (0.020, 0.025), $p<0.001$). $LAeq_{(1-min)}$ and LFN both had negative interaction effect estimates with wind direction on ln(PNC) outcomes in these models.

4.3.1.3 Effect Modifications of Wind Direction from Local Roadways

While impact sector winds originated from the direction of local roadways, the effect estimates for impact sector interactions in models including noise parameters and temporal factors all had negative associations with ln(PNC). Exceptions to this include VLFN: Impact_Wind_Road in Chelsea in a model with LFN and time of day (Model 8: $\beta = 0.012$, 95% ci (0.01, 0.015), $p<0.001$);

Impact_Wind_Road:VLFN in Roxbury in a model with LAeq($_{1\text{-min}}$) and time of day (Model 9: $\beta = 0.013$, 95% ci (0.008, 0.019), $p<0.001$), and LAeq: Impact_Wind_Road also in Roxbury in a model with LFN and time of day (Model 10: $\beta = 0.014$, 95% ci (0.007, 0.022), $p<0.001$).

4.3.1.4 Effect Modifications of Wind Direction from Roxbury Bus Station

Models 9 and 10 evaluate interactions of noise covariates and impact sector winds from the direction of the Nubian Square MBTA (T) bus station, located 75 m. WNW of the Roxbury site. Bus traffic from this terminal was approximately 250 buses/day during the study period April -September 2016 (*mbta.com*). We found that the interaction of LAeq: Wind_Impact_Bus and VLFN: Wind_Impact_Bus were directionally opposite and of similar magnitude in a model with both noise covariates and time of day. Respectively, Model 9: $\beta = 0.015$, 95% ci (0.01, 0.02), $p<0.001$; $\beta = -0.014$, 95% ci (-0.02, -0.01), $p<0.001$.

Lastly, in Model 10, which included LAeq($_{1\text{-min}}$) and LFN noise measures, time of day and wind impact sector interactions with noise covariates, we found that the interaction of wind impact sector from the Roxbury bus station with LAeq($_{1\text{-min}}$) and LFN were directionally opposite; their effect estimates increased in magnitude 185% in the positive direction as follows: LAeq: Wind_Impact_Bus effect estimate $\beta = -0.014$, 95% ci (-0.02, -0.01), $p<0.001$, and LFN: Wind_Impact_Bus effect estimate $\beta = 0.034$, 95% ci (0.027, 0.041), $p<0.001$ (**Table 5S**, Supplementary Materials, Appendix 2).

4.4   Wind-Robust Model

Based on our findings, a wind-robust model, controlling for impact sector wind direction and including an interaction term for wind speed would take the form:

Eq(1): ln(PNC) = β_o + β_1*VLFN (dB) + β_2*LFN (dB) + β_3*[LFN*(wind_speed (km/hr)] + e

Testing this proposed model for wind direction controlled from Logan Airport, an impact sector common to both sites (5% of all wind direction readings during our study), and cited by Hudda et al. (2016) and Simon et al. (2017) as a wind direction contributory to increased PNC to both Chelsea and Roxbury, for median values of VLFN (dB), LFN (dB) and wind speed (km/hr), this proposed model yields ln(PNC) = 3.29 -0.027(62.7 dB VLFN)+0.12(70.6 dB LFN) -0.0001(70.6 dB*12.9 km/hr) or ln(PNC) = 9.87. Exponentiating both sides results in a PNC concentration = **19,270** particles/cm^3.

When tested for wind direction controlled from local roads, representing road traffic at both sites (11% of all wind direction readings during our study), for median values of VLFN (dB), LFN (dB) and wind speed (km/hr), this proposed model yields: ln(PNC) ~ 5.48 -0.012(64.2 dB VLFN) +0.072(70.6 dB LFN) -0.0002(70.6 dB*16.7 km/hr) or ln(PNC) ~ 9.58. Exponentiating both sides results in a PNC concentration = **14,512** particles/cm^3.

Stratified by site (Chelsea==0; Roxbury ==1), controlled for wind impact sector==airport (v. all other wind impact sectors (i.e. wind impact sector airport==0)), and also modeling median values for VLFN, LFN and wind speed, we found similar results. Our proposed wind robust model predicted 11,389 particles/cm^3 for Chelsea wind impact sector=airport v. 8,111 particles/cm^3 for all other wind impact sectors, a 1.4-fold PNC concentration increase from the airport sector. For Roxbury, the model predicted 23,717 particles/cm^3 for Roxbury wind impact sector=airport v. 16,579 particles/cm^3 for all other wind impact sectors, also a 1.4-fold PNC concentration increase. The effect estimate for VLFN in the Roxbury model, however was not significant ($p>0.05$).

Our proposed wind-robust models are supported by work from Hudda et al., which found that the annual (2014) average impact-sector PNC from Logan Airport was 2-fold higher than the average for all other wind directions in Chelsea [35 000 ± 75% (average ± relative standard deviation) compared to 18 000 ± 69% particles cm−3], and 1.33 fold higher in Roxbury [28 000 ± 54% (average ± relative standard deviation) compared to 21 000 ± 65% particles cm−3] (Hudda, et al., 2016), and further supported by

Simon et al. (2017) who found that during SSE winds at Chelsea, average PNC was approximately twice the average for all other wind directions (Simon et al., 2017).

Figure 2 presents hourly average baseline PNC roses (normalized to the maximum) for the two sites for this study period (April -September, 2016).

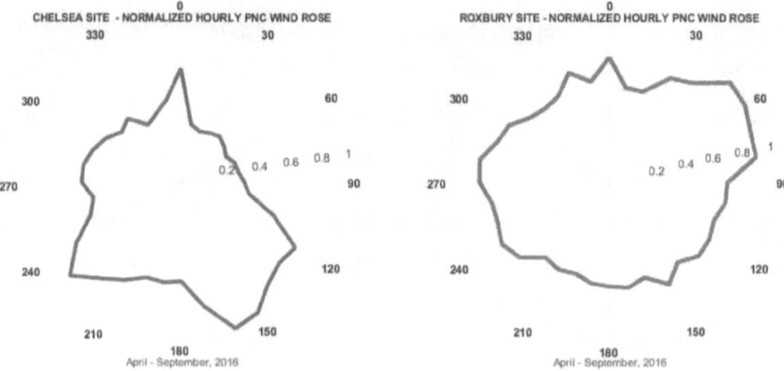

Figure 2 Hourly Average Baseline PNC Roses (Normalized to the Maximum)

The PNC roses in **Fig. 2** are similar to those presented by Hudda et al. (2016) for the same locations and were prepared to the same specifications as in that study. We additionally plotted noise-PNC wind roses (**Figure 3**) to assess the contribution of combined noise levels (LAeq($_{1-min}$)) and noise frequencies to PNC concentrations by wind direction. We additionally created heatmaps of mean PNC concentration (**Figure 4**) for 1-min averages of LAeq and noise frequencies. Heatmaps show mean PNC concentrations (#/cm^3) by wind impact sector for various noise measures, grouped by quartiles. Colorbars in all figure panels (**Figs. 3, 4**) show PNC concentrations (particles/cm^3).

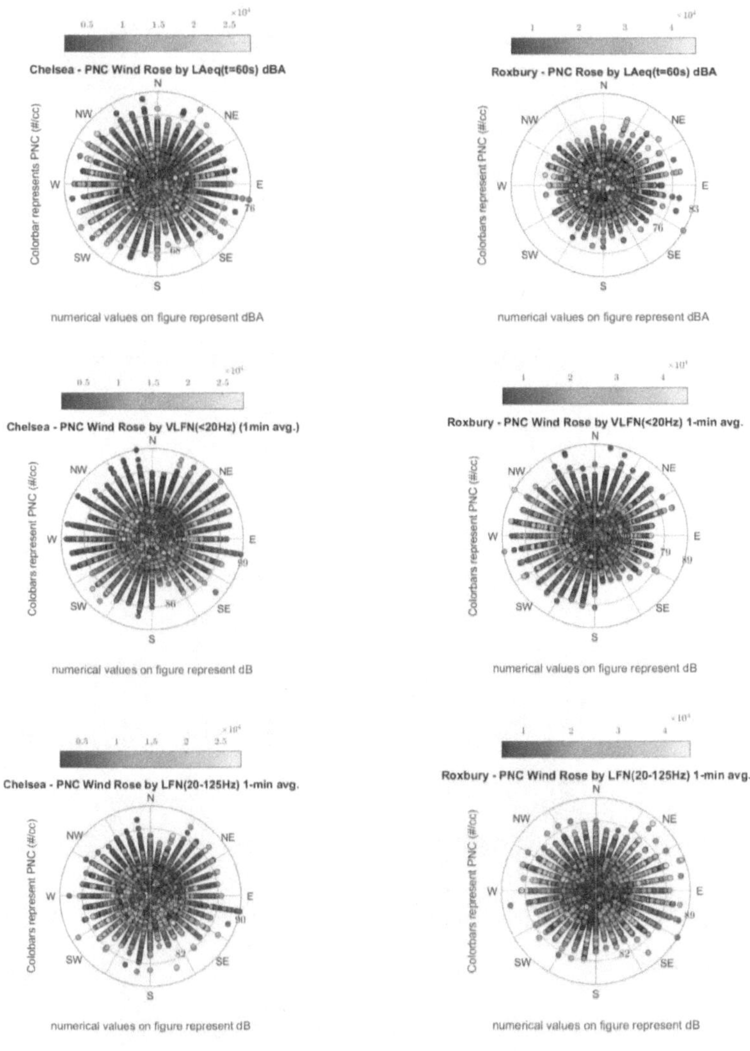

Figure 3 PNC Wind Roses for Noise Covariates (left panels = Chelsea; right panels = Roxbury)

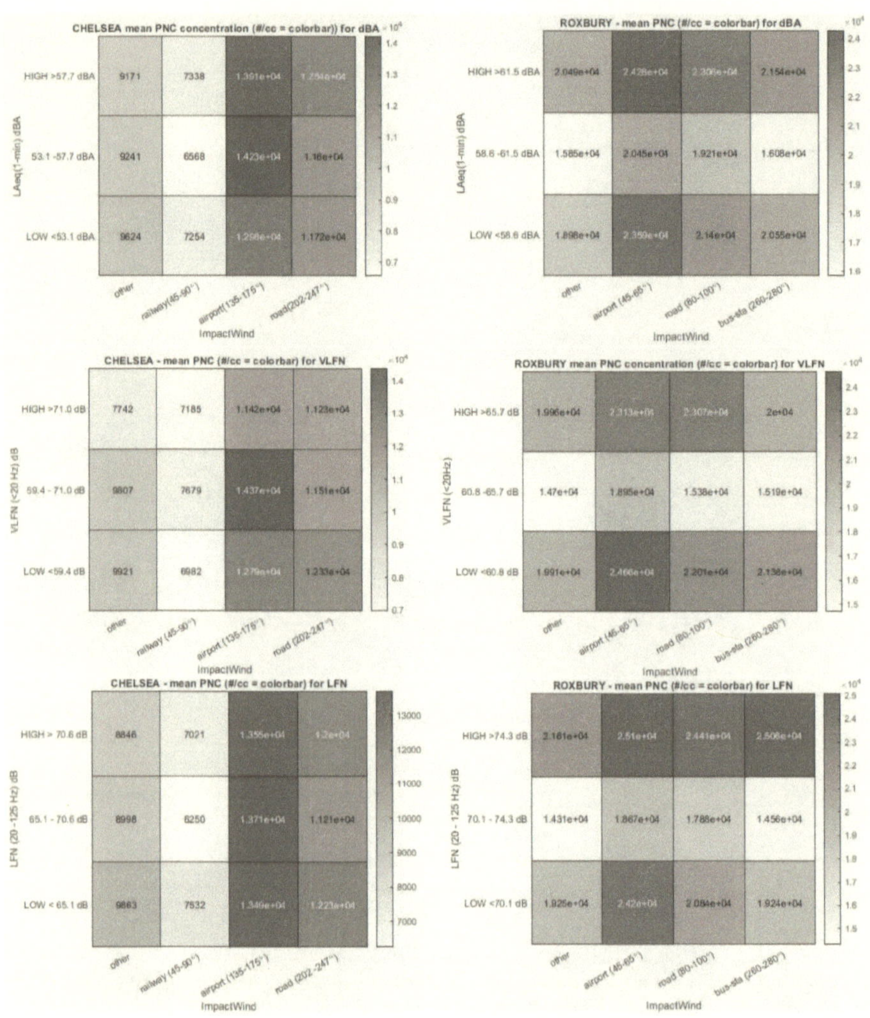

Figure 4 Heatmaps of PNC Concentration (#/cc) for Noise Measures by Impact Wind Sector
(left panels = Chelsea; right panels = Roxbury)

4.4.1   Model Validation Support

To support validation of our models, we plotted time series for each site on selected dates

controlled for transportation source (**Figure 5(a)(b)(c)**). Time series transportation source data were

either visually confirmed (Roxbury, **Fig. 5** right) or audibly logged from .mp3 sound recordings and

verified by Logan Airport flight take-off and landing schedules or MBTA train schedules. Each boxed

region represents dates/times when the impact wind direction (Wind Dir) originates from the same

category as the Source, identified by black dots in the figures, which represent a single event (i.e. –

vehicle passing the microphone).

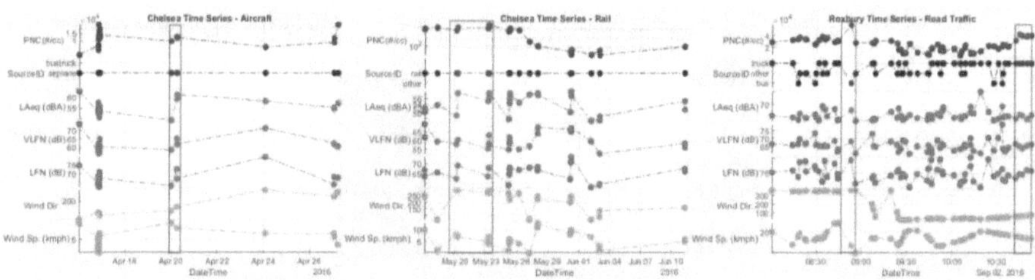

Fig. 5 Time Series Plots for Selected Dates by Transportation Source

For selected April 2016 Chelsea aircraft noise events (**Fig. 5(a)**, left), shown within the

rectangular boxed region (April 20, 2016) there was a 22.5% increase in PNC concentrations (9,670 to

11,850 particles/cm^3); a concomitant increase in LAeq($_{1-min}$) levels by +11.8 dBA from 49.2 dBA to 61.1

dBA; VLFN increased +3.3 dB from 58.5 dB to 61.8 dB; and LFN increased +3.6 dB from 63.7 to 67.3

dB, while wind direction shifted from 90° to 135° – to within the Logan Airport wind impact sector. Wind

speed decreased slightly, from 11 to 9 km/hr during this event. These observations support our findings

from Model 7 (**Table 5S**, Supplementary Materials, Appendix 2), which predicted that during impact

sector winds from the direction of Logan Airport (wind direction SE: 135 -175°), both LAeq($_{1-min}$) and

LFN had positive interaction effect estimates with wind direction on *ln*(PNC) outcome.

The highest concentrations of PNC from identified rail transportation noise sources (trains) in Chelsea for selected study dates May 17-June 11, 2016 (**Fig. 5(b)**, center) occurred May 20 -23, 2016 while winds were from 270° to 292°, placing the Chelsea monitoring site downwind of the MBTA rail line and local roads (Broadway, **Fig. 1**). PNC concentrations reached 24,900 particles/cm^3 during these impact sector winds (rectangular boxed region), and with each train noise event recorded LAeq($_{1-min}$) increased 3 -10 dB(A); VLFN increased 2 -5 dB; and LFN increased 4 -8 dBA Wind speeds were relatively light 1 -8 km/hr during these events.

In **Fig. 5** (c) (right), PNC concentrations increased more than 2-fold from a previous reading of 29,900 particles/cm^3 and peaked at 71,900 particles/cm^3 during a bus transit event at 09:00am in Roxbury on September 2, 2016. LAeq($_{1-min}$) increased +7.7 dBA from 58.0 to 65.7 dBA; VLFN increased +5 dB from 63.1 to 68.1 dB; and LFN increased +6.1 dB 73.3 to 79.4 dB. Wind was consistently from the north (360°) during and prior to this event, which was not from the direction of the MBTA bus terminal (260° -280°). Wind speeds, which were high-to-moderate during this event, decreased from 22.2 km/hr to 16.7 km/hr (75th percentile was 20.3 km/hr).

The additional rectangular boxed region in **Fig. 5(c)** (right), after 10:30am, represents increased PNC concentrations as wind steadies from the roadway wind impact sector 20-75°, during which PNC increased 3-fold from a baseline 14,000 particles /cm^3 to 42,500 particles/cm^3. LAeq($_{1-min}$) ,VLFN and LFN varied minimally (+/- 3 dB). Wind speeds remained steady, at a moderate 18-19 km/hr. It is likely that the localized spikes and increased trends in PNC (**Fig. 3**(c) right) may be due to buses and trucks travelling roughly N-S along Harrison Ave (**Fig. 1**) recorded by both the sound meters and PNC monitors at the Roxbury site.

4.5   General Discussion

4.5.1   Key findings

Based upon 5-months of continuous noise and PNC sampling at two urban sites in Greater Boston, MA, we found that LAeq(time), VLFN and LFN are associated with *In*(PNC) concentrations, mediated by wind direction and wind speeds. VLFN imparts slight negative effects on *In*(PNC), depending on wind speed and impact sector wind direction (airport, roadways, rail lines, bus station). In models with either VLFN or LFN we found that LAeq(time) (dBA) has positive effects on *In*(PNC). A novel, wind-robust model was developed using lower noise frequencies (f<125Hz) as transportation-source proxies, interacting with wind speed to estimate PNC concentrations from impact sector wind directions. The predicted model results were supported by PNC and meteorological data measurements and analyses conducted by others at the same two sites (Hudda et al., 2016, Simon et al. 2017).

4.5.2 Synthesis with previous research

Despite extensive previous study of spatiotemporal factors' effect on variation in transportation noise, links between transportation noise emissions and meteorology-mediated emissions of PNC have not been well defined (Can, Rademaker, et al., 2011). Adding to the complexity of these relationships is the fact that noise and air pollution are often correlated due to shared sources (Poulsen et al., Lancet, 2023). According to the US EPA (2007) motor vehicles, especially those powered by diesel engines, have often been cited as a leading source of ambient UFP emissions and of deleterious effects on human health (Ris, C., 2007).

Waye (2004) affirms that low frequency noise (LFN), defined in their work as 20Hz-200Hz, is associated with transportation sources, including trucks, diesel buses, trains and aircraft (Waye, K.P., 2004). Ascari et al. (2014) presents a broader definition of LFN as 10Hz -250Hz, and attributes the source to diesel engine and transportation vehicles (Ascari, et al., 2015). Sound below 20 Hz is generally termed infrasound (Alves, 2020) and while it may subjectively be considered a component of low-frequency noise, it is inaudible (Bergland, 1996).

A literature search of international research on LFN from motor vehicles has revealed that the major frequency content of motor vehicle emission in terms of one third octave bands is in the range of 63 Hz to 125 Hz depending on vehicle speed and engine size (Roberts, 2010). Other sources of low frequency noise and infrasound are produced by machinery, both rotational and reciprocating, and all forms of transport. Typical sources include pumps, compressors, diesel engines, aircraft and fans (Roberts, 2010). Of these VLFN and LFN sources, diesel engines in particular are also sources of UFP emissions. These also include commuter trains (Jeong, et al., 2017, airport-related emissions (Hudda et al., EST, 2016), and heavy-duty diesel trucks and buses, which typically emit 10 times as many particles as a gasoline-engine car (Morawska et al., 2005; Ritovski et al., 2006).

Research on noise exposure to urban cyclists in Belgium has shown that engine-related traffic noise encountered along the bicyclist's route is a valid indicator of black carbon (BC), yet BC does not correlate with noise expressed as A-weighted equivalent sound pressure levels (LAeq($_{time}$)) (Dekoninck, L.; Botteldooren, D.; et al., 2013). Dekoninck and European colleagues (2016) emphasize that the correlation between noise and particulate matter exposure is complex, noting that noise measurements contain spectral information that is highly relevant to improve this correlation, and specific noise indicators could be derived for this purpose. Dekoninck et al. add that simultaneous noise and BC and UFP measurements add significant value to the quality of air pollution models.

A significant potential exists for developing a standard tool or model to assess combined exposure of traffic related air and noise pollution to facilitate health related studies (Khan, J., et al. 2018). Studies employing deterministic modelling to study exposures to both covariates reported moderate positive to slightly higher positive air-noise correlations (Örgen and Molnar, 2014; Sørensen et al., 2012). Although deterministic models have been criticized in the literature, specifically that the majority fail to predict extreme concentrations (Khare and Sharma, 2002), they are considered powerful and flexible tools (Khan, J., et al. 2018).

4.5.3   Effect Modifications of Meteorology

Impact sector winds were important determinants of *In*(PNC), with the strongest positive effects from winds from the direction of Logan Airport and from the road and railway at Chelsea. Patton et al., (2015) found that wind-direction sectors that included the airport as a possible upwind source were a significant explanatory variable for PNC in communities located 4–8 km north-northwest (NNW) – south-southwest (SSW) of the airport in Boston (Patton et al., 2015).

Supporting our findings, Hudda et al. (2016) found that relatively high PNCs were observed (2014 average was 22 000 ± 53% particles/cm^3) during southwesterly winds when highway US1 (2.6×10^4 vehicles/ day) and local streets and intersections were upwind of the Chelsea site. Hudda et al. (2016) also observed coincident concentration spikes of gaseous pollutants and PNCs when winds were from the direction of busy intersections in the vicinity of the Roxbury site (southeast and west), with the highest of the daily averages at Roxbury site (>50 000 particles /cm^3) coincident with northwest winds in winter, reflecting contributions from traffic-related emissions (Hudda et al., 2016).

In Roxbury interaction effects of impact sector winds from Harrison Ave. and from the Nubian Square bus station had significant positive associations with *In*(PNC) for VLFN (road) and LFN and LAeq($_{1\text{-min}}$) (bus station). We hypothesize that this nearly three-fold increase effect is due to particulate matter from LFN-emitting diesel bus engine exhausts reaching the Roxbury monitoring site carried by impact sector winds from the West (260° -280°). These compass bearings were identified by Hudda et al. (2016) as a comparable impact sector wind direction v. Logan Airport for equivalent mean hourly average PNC concentrations (particles/cm^3) at the Roxbury site (Hudda et al., 2016).

Simon et al. (2017) additionally note that the location of the Boston (Roxbury) central-site monitor is in a highly-trafficked area (i.e., at grade and 75 m from the Dudley Square bus station) compared to most of the Boston residential sites. Simon et al. (2017) used the EPA-STN Roxbury site, a secure, centrally-located site >1500 m from I-93, which was likely influenced by bus emissions when winds were from the 225-315° sector.

Figures 3 and **4** show noise levels for various wind directions and impact sectors, colored by PNC concentrations (particles/cm^3). PNC wind roses in **Figure 3(a)** suggest that higher dBA (LAeq($_{1-min}$)) levels are indicative of higher PNC concentrations from the local roadways (westerly direction) in Chelsea (left figure) and more widely distributed PNC concentrations from the directions of the bus station, airport and local roads in Roxbury (right figure). **Figure 3(b)** shows a clear spike in PNC concentrations from the direction of Logan Airport (135 -175°) while VLFN dB levels are elevated in Chelsea (left figure); the bus station remains a transport source of PNC with higher VLFN dB levels in Roxbury (right figure). LFN wind roses **(Fig. 3(c))** appear similar to dBA wind roses, with wider PNC distributions by wind direction at both sites.

Figure 4 presents heatmaps of mean PNC concentrations (particles/cm^3) for quartiles of noise levels. (<25th percentile = Q1; IQR = 25th- 75th percentile; and >75th percentile, dBA and dB values shown on **Fig. 4**) for impact wind sectors as previously identified in this study as known sources of PNC (airport, railway, roadways). The highest mean PNC concentrations occur from wind impact sectors from Logan Airport for all noise measures at both sites. Secondary to this are elevated mean PNC concentrations from the roadways (both sites) and from the bus station wind impact sector in Roxbury. Taken together, **Figures 3** and **4** indicate that impact wind directions from Logan Airport, local roadways and the Roxbury bus station result in the highest mean PCN concentrations, with variation in the PNC concentrations occurring at differing levels of noise measures.

Of the other meteorological covariates modeled - temperature, humidity (%) and wind speed - only wind speed==HI (75th percentile) more strongly affected model results for various noise covariate associations with *ln*(PNC). Hudda et al. (2016) found that during impact-sector winds, the highest PNCs were observed during 25–35 km/hr winds at Chelsea and 30–50 km/hr winds at Roxbury. The highest

PNCs for winds from other directions were observed during calm to <10 km/hr wind speeds. (Hudda et al., 2016).

A study in Montreal by Weichenthal et al. (2015) found that wind speed had a negative effect estimate on mean UFP concentration (particles/cm^3) (β = -1534, 95% ci (-1912, -1156)) in a linear regression model, and cited that ambient temperature and wind speed are known to be important predictors of temporal variations in ambient UFP concentrations. The Montreal study additionally presented a model for the natural logarithm of ambient UFPs, which explained a similar proportion of the variance in ambient UFP concentrations vs. mean UFP (not log transformed) concentrations (Weichenthal, S. et al., 2015).

We hypothesize that under high wind speed conditions, LFN may not be a significant predictor of *ln*(PNC) and VLFN is a poor predictor of *ln*(PNC). Under light to moderate wind speeds (upper quartile), LFN is a stronger positive predictor and VLFN may be a directionally negative predictor of *ln*(PNC) depending upon site and wind direction, although VLFN is moderately correlated to wind speed (r=0.4 - 0.65).

4.5.4   Temporal Factors Affecting PNC

Time of day was included in our models as a temporal covariate as Day==0700-2300hrs; Night==2300 -0700hrs, and had significant positive effect estimates on *ln*(PNC) outcomes. Simon et al. (2017) found that overnight PNC in Chelsea was substantially lower compared to daytime concentrations and noted an increase in Chelsea PNC was observed during the evening rush hour period, and especially during south-southeast (SSE) winds (Simon, et al. 2017).

4.5.5   Assessment of Confounding

Two-pollutant models of noise and air pollution exposures have attempted to disentangle which factors are independent risk factors for health outcomes and quantify their contribution to the total environmental burden (Poulsen et al., 2023). Tetreault et al. (2013) affirm that more studies using pollution indicators specific to road traffic are needed to properly assess if noise and air pollution are subjected to confounding (Tetreault, L., et al., 2013).

Significant moderate correlations between 1-min averages of PNC and noise imply that in epidemiological studies of health effects of air pollution during traffic exposures, modest confounding may occur if noise is ignored (Boogard et al., 2009). Because correlations are moderate, statistical methods can be used to indentify the potential independent effects of air pollution and noise, provided both are monitored (ibid).

Goldberg et al. (2008) describe the necessary conditions for confounding in time-series studies as (1) the potential confounder is causally related to the outcome and (2) exposures to the pollutant of interest and the potential confounder co-vary (Goldberg et al., 2008). In our study, noise and wind speed could be confounded since both variables are related to the outcome of PNC concentration. We evaluated confounding effects of wind speed on noise in our wind-robust models (**Table 4**). Models of dBA (LAeq($_{1-min}$)) showed a difference of 200% in the β-coefficient, directionally negative (airport wind impact sector), when wind speed (km/hr) was added to the model.

β-coefficients differed from 39% directionally positive (airport wind impact sectors) to 500% directionally negative (roadway impact sectors), when wind speed (km/hr) was added to VLFN-only models. LFN-only models β-coefficients differed only 5% directionally positive from both airport and road wind impact sectors when wind speed was added to those models. For combined VLFN+LFN models, β-coefficients differed <1% for LFN directionally positive and from 5% to 25% directionally negative for VLFN upon addition of wind speed (results in Appendix 2, **Table 6S**, Supplementary Tables).

We conclude that wind speed and VLFN are confounded in models predicting *ln*(PNC) in our study. Wind speed and its interactions with LFN can be modeled with VLFN in the same models with only small changes in model β-coefficients for VLFN. We found no confounding effects of wind speed with LFN, and generally higher R^2 values and lower AIC values for lower freqeuncy noise (<125Hz) models v. dBA models.

4.5.6 Wind Robust Model Discussion

Our proposed wind-robust model, controlling for wind impact sector (direction) has good agreement with prior work conducted at the same sites and may be valid to predict average or median PNC values, based on median noise measures of VLFN (dB) and LFN (dB), with interactions of LFN and median wind speeds (km/hr). The proposed model may not be as strong a predictor for individual noise-PNC events such as PNC emissions from a single source of road traffic pollution (e.g. buses, trucks).

We found that models comprised of lower noise-frequencies (VLFN, LFN) and their interactions with wind speed, controlled for wind impact sectors from Logan airport performed better (AIC: 9.6E3; R^2= 0.27) at predicting ln(PNC) than a dBA-only model with LAeq($_{1\text{-min}}$) and a dBA:wind speed interaction model (AIC: 1.03E4; R^2=0.16)(**Table 4**).

Similar results were found for models predicting ln(PNC) with wind impact sectors from local roadways (**Table 4**). Lower noise-frequency (VLFN, LFN) models and their interactions with wind speed also performed better (AIC: 1.77E4; R^2= 0.22) at predicting ln(PNC) than a dBA-only model (AIC: 1.87E4; R^2= 0.15). Additional models of C-weighted (nearly independent of frequency) minus A-weighted decibels, LCeq-LAeq(24-hr) when paired with dBA and wind speed were not significant predictors (p>0.05) of ln(PNC).

There exists no standard or harmonized tool in the scientific literature for modeling both exposures to noise and air pollution simultaneously (Khan, J. et al., 2018). The novelty of our wind-robust model is its use of lower noise frequencies as transportation-source proxies, interacting with wind speed to estimate PNC concentrations from impact sector wind directions. Other work in our study areas by Patton et al. (2015), Hudda et al. (2016) and Simon et al. (2017) did not include noise as a covariate in their PNC models or correlation analyses.

4.5.7 Study strengths and weaknesses

This study, encompassing five months of ambient noise monitoring in two locations is markedly different in its length and depth of noise measures and meteorological measurements from previous studies. Our dataset is available for other researchers as a .txt file possessing rich metrics of dBA and 1/3 octave bands, encompassing some 1 billion readings. Our data are currently being evaluated for implementing a machine-learning modeling approach. This will help further define spatiotemporal differences in both loudness and noise frequencies classified by source (e.g. truck, bus, rail, aircraft) and source impacts on PNC concentrations mediated by meterology.

Although we collected data across two seasons (late-Spring through late-Summer), we did not capture Winter seasonality to assess the previously reported inverse relationship between ambient temperature and UFPs (Weichenthal, S. et al. 2015). Indeed Simon et al. (2017) found that PNC was highest during winter (December-February) and lowest during summer (June-August) with median winter concentrations up to a factor of two higher than median summer concentrations in Boston (inclusive of the Roxbury site), with similar temporal trends in the Chelsea study area (Hudda et al., 2016; Simon, et al. 2017).

The use of one omni-directional sensor (microphone) at each site and therefore being unable to determine directionality of noise or perform separation of VLFN (infrasound) from wind noise is a limitation in this study, although we did perform statistical analyses of wind speed and wind direction impacts on lower frequencies to ascertain their confounding effects.

4.5.8 Implications for future research

A related area of focus from this study is use of visibility as a variable of interest for correlations with PNC. While we found very weak to weak (Spearman's r=0.06 to r=0.29) positive correlations between PNC (particles/cm^3) and visibility (km), stratifying by wind speed (see Section 4.2), the literature suggests that slow-moving air masses—and therefore stagnant conditions—facilitate the build-up of accumulation mode particles (100 -1000nm particle size), resulting in the poorest visibility (i-Hao Young, Chih-Sheng Hsu, et al. 2023). A study conducted in Taiwan applied positive matrix factorization (PMF) to identify the sources of size-resolved submicrometer (10–1000 nm) particles and quantify their contributions to impaired visibility based on the particle number size distributions (PNSDs), aerosol light extinction, other pollutants and meteorological parameters (i-Hao Young, et al. 2023). Hopke et al. (2022) identified 55 peer-reviewed journal articles on the source apportionment of particles contributing to PNSDs in 102 locations/time periods. Those studies, however, did not further investigate the link between the PMF and atmospheric visibility (Hopke, P. et al., 2022). Futher reasearch correlating visibility and PNC is warranted.

4.5.9   Implications on the regulatory process

The present paper relies on frequency (f, Hz) as a proxy for tranportation noise source, with diesel-emitting sources linked to frequencies <125Hz as a proxy for Low Frequency Noise. Studies focused on the health effects of noise instead generally express noise levels as a function of A-weighted decibels (dBA). A-weighting has a long history in health studies and provides a consistent metric to aid comparison between studies, yet A-weighting significantly de-emphasizes low frequency noise. The World Health Organization (WHO) has specifically warned against the limitations associated with reliance on A-weighting in health studies, and states that noise with a large proportion of low-frequency components 'may increase considerably the effects on health' (Berglund et al., 1996).

While dBA captures time-weighted sound pressure levels, such as $LAeq_{(time)}$, it may be linked to sources that do not emit air pollutants, such as neighborhood noise, or music, both of which are omnipresent in modern urban societies. Work by Lee, N et al., (2022) also in Greater Boston, notes that of the types of community noise, entertainment and leisure are influence both urban noise perception (perceived loudness) and high frequency sound levels (Lee, N., Levy, J., et al. (2022)).

A lengthy body of literature, much of which is previously cited in this book, links VLFN and LFN

components of UEN to transportation sources, including trucks, diesel buses, trains and aircraft (Waye,

K.P., (2004))(Ascari et al. (2014); each are known sources of UFP emissions. One caveat is that

infrasound and low freqeuncy noise sources may also include pumps, compressors and fans (Roberts,

2010). These may not be UFP-emitting devices.

One immediate effect of the long history of A-weighted noise monitoring is that there is an

abundance of dBA noise data being collected across the world principally at airports. Regulatory

implications could involve collection of flat-weighted 1/3-octave band noise frequency data in addition to

dBA at airport locations to facilitate further exposure studies in capturing and assessing the contributions

of VLFN and LFN to the soundscape of airport environs.

4.6   Recommendations

Based on favorable results of our proposed wind-robust model, we recommend replicating the

model in other locations for assessment of the model's generalizability. Possible locations could be those

in which we have active collaborations, such as Cincinnati, OH, where the author has previously

collaborated with researchers conducting a joint noise and UFP personal exposure study (Leaffer, et al.,

2019). We also recommend replicating our wind robust model in Los Angeles, CA where one of our Tufts

University collaborators conducted a study on long-range (10 km downwind) effects of PNC emissions

from aviation emisions (Hudda, N. et al. 2014). Historical noise data from the airport may be useful in

such a study.

5.0   Conclusions

This study explores the complex interaction between noise and ultrafine particles (UFP<100nm

diameter), emphasizing the potential improvement in correlation through a richer set of noise indicators.

Simultaneous environmental noise and PNC (a proxy for UFP) measurements are explored to enhance the quality of air pollution models and examine the association of transportation-related noise frequencies on PNC. Additionally, the impact of wind parameters on the noise-PNC association is investigated.

Over a 5-month period, noise and PNC were measured at two urban sites in Greater Boston, Massachusetts, burdened with multiple environmental noise and air pollution sources. The study evaluated if loudness and noise frequencies, identified through 1/3-octave band spectral analysis, correlate with PNC . Moderately correlated (r<0.65) noise and meteorological covariates were modeled by multivariate regression. Models of A-weighted (dBA) noise and lower noise frequencies (f<125 Hz) were chosen to capture the impact of diesel engine emissions as a source of importance.

We found that VLFN (<20Hz) imparts slight negative effects on log-transformed PNC, depending on wind speed and impact sector wind direction (airport, roadways, rail lines, bus station). In contrast, LFN imparts positive effects of a similar magnitude. In VLFN or LFN models, sound pressure levels, measured as $LAeq_{(time)}$ (dBA) have positive effects on ln(PNC).

A wind-robust model, controlling for impact sector wind direction and including a wind speed interaction term was developed and validated. The proposed wind-robust model aligns well with prior research conducted at the same sites, which did not consider noise as a covariate. It may effectively predict average or median PNC values based on median noise measures of VLFN and LFN, considering interactions with median wind speeds. However, the model's strength as a predictor for individual (e.g., bus, truck) noise-PNC events may be limited.

6.0   References

1. Goines, L., & Hagler, L. (2007). Noise pollution: a modern plague. South Med J, 100(3), 287- 94).
2. EMEP, EEA, and EEA Air Pollutant Emission Inventory Guidebook. Technical Guidance to Prepare National Emission Inventories. No. 12. EEA Technical Report, (2013).
3. Health Effects Institute. Panel on the Health Effects of Traffic-Related Air Pollution. "Traffic-related air pollution: a critical review of the literature on emissions, exposure, and health effects." (2010).
4. United Nations, (2022).
5. P. De Vos, A. Van Beek, (2011)
6. Baliatsas, Christos, et al. "Health effects from low-frequency noise and infrasound in the general population: Is it time to listen? A systematic review of observational studies." Science of the Total Environment 557 (2016): 163-169.
7. Hudda, N., et al. "Aviation emissions impact ambient ultrafine particle concentrations in the greater Boston area." Environmental science & technology 50.16 (2016): 8514-8521.
8. Health Effects Institute (HEI). HEI Perspectives. Vol. 3. HEI; Boston, MA: (2013). HEI Review Panel on Ultrafine Particles. Understanding the Health Effects of Ambient Ultrafine Particles
9. Allen, et al., (The spatial relationship between traffic-generated air pollution and noise in 2 US cities, NIH, Environ Res., (2009).
10. Ross Z, Kheirbek I, Clougherty JE, Ito K, Matte T, Markowitz S, Eisl H: Noise, air pollution and traffic: Continuous measurement and correlation at a high-traffic location in New York City. Environ Res (2011).
11. Can, A., Rademaker, M., et al., Correlation analysis of noise and ultrafine particle counts in a street canyon. Science of the Total Environment, 409(3), 564-572, (2011).
12. Khan, Jibran, et al., "Road traffic air and noise pollution exposure assessment–A review of tools and techniques." Science of the total environment 634 (2018): 661-676.
13. Dekoninck, L., De Coensel, B., & Int Panis, L. (2016, August). Spectral noise measurements supply instantaneous traffic information for multidisciplinary mobility and traffic related projects. In INTER-NOISE and NOISE-CON Congress and Conference Proceedings (Vol. 253, No. 1, pp. 6934-6940). Institute of Noise Control Engineering.
14. Walker, Erica D., et al., "Descriptive characterization of sound levels in an environmental justice city before and during a global pandemic." Environmental Research" 199 (2021).
15. Mass DOT, (2016)
16. mbta.com, (2016)
17. Massport.com, (2016)
18. City of Boston, (2015)
19. Protocol for a Sleep Study (PARTNER, Sleep Study #25 Acoustics System), (2014)
20. Logan Airport, Boston historical weather records (KBOS)
21. B. Goelzer, C.H. Hansen, G.A. Sehrndt, Fundamentals of Acoustics, Occupational Exposure to Noise: Evaluation, Prevention and Control, Bremerhaven: Wirtschaftsverlag N.W (2001)
22. Leaffer, Douglas J., et al., "Long-term measurement study of urban environmental low frequency noise." Journal of Exposure Science & Environmental Epidemiology (2023): 1-13.

23. Simon, Matthew C., et al., "Comparisons of traffic-related ultrafine particle number concentrations measured in two urban areas by central, residential, and mobile monitoring." Atmospheric Environment 169 (2017): 113-127.

24. Boogaard, Hanna, et al., "Exposure to ultrafine and fine particles and noise during cycling and driving in 11 Dutch cities." Atmospheric Environment 43.27 (2009): 4234-4242.

25. Ragettli, Martina S., et al., "Statistical modeling of the spatial variability of environmental noise levels in Montreal, Canada, using noise measurements and land use characteristics." Journal of Exposure Science & Environmental Epidemiology 26.6 (2016): 597-605.

26. Patton, Allison P., et al., "Transferability and generalizability of regression models of ultrafine particles in urban neighborhoods in the Boston area." Environmental science & technology 49.10 (2015): 6051-6060.

27. the Mathworks nd

28. i-Hao Young, Chih-Sheng Hsu, et al., Sources, transport, and visibility impact of ambient submicrometer particle number size distributions in an urban area of central Taiwan, Science of The Total Environment, Volume 856, Part 2, (2023).

29. Poulsen, Aslak H., et al., "Concomitant exposure to air pollution, green space, and noise and risk of stroke: a cohort study from Denmark." The Lancet Regional Health–Europe 31 (2023).

30. Ris, Charles. "US EPA health assessment for diesel engine exhaust: a review." Inhalation toxicology 19.sup1 (2007): 229-239.

31. Waye, K. Persson. "Effects of low frequency noise on sleep." Noise and health 6.23 (2004): 87-91.

32. Ascari, Elena, et al., "Low frequency noise impact from road traffic according to different noise prediction methods." Science of the total environment 505 (2015): 658-669.

33. Araújo Alves, Juliana, et al., "Low-frequency noise and its main effects on human health—A review of the literature between 2016 and 2019." Applied Sciences 10.15 (2020): 5205.

34. Berglund B, Hassmen P, Job RS. Sources and effects of low-frequency noise. J Acoustical Soc Am. (1996);99:2985–3002.

35. Nina F. Lee, Jonathan I. Levy, Marcos Luna, Erica D. Walker, Spatial and sociodemographic determinants of community loudness perception, Applied Acoustics, Volume 186, (2022).

36. Roberts, C. , Proceedings of 20th International Congress on Acoustics, ICA 2010 23-27 August 2010, Sydney, Australia ICA 2010 "Low Frequency Noise from Transportation Sources".

37. Jeong, Cheol-Heon, Alison Traub, and Greg J. Evans. "Exposure to ultrafine particles and black carbon in diesel-powered commuter trains." Atmospheric Environment 155 (2017): 46-52.

38. Morawska, Lidia, et al., "Experimental study of the deposition of combustion aerosols in the human respiratory tract." Journal of Aerosol Science 36.8 (2005): 939-957.

39. Ristovski, Z. D., et al., "Influence of diesel fuel sulfur on nanoparticle emissions from city buses." Environmental science & technology 40.4 (2006): 1314-1320.

40. Dekoninck, Luc, Dick Botteldooren, and Luc Int Panis. "An instantaneous spatiotemporal model to predict a bicyclist's Black Carbon exposure based on mobile noise measurements." Atmospheric Environment 79 (2013): 623-631.

41. Ögren, Mikael, and Peter Molnar. "Correlation between Noise and NOx in Gothenburg 1975-2010." ISEE Conference Abstracts 26. Vol. 2014. No. 1. 2014.

42. Sørensen, Mette, et al., "Road traffic noise and incident myocardial infarction: a prospective cohort study." PloS one 7.6 (2012): e39283.

43. Khare, M., and P. Sharma. "Vehicular Emission Modelling." (2002).

44. Weichenthal, Scott, et al., "Long-term exposure to ambient ultrafine particles and respiratory disease incidence in in Toronto, Canada: a cohort study." Environmental Health 16 (2017): 1-11.

45. Tétreault, Louis-François, Stéphane Perron, and Audrey Smargiassi. "Cardiovascular health, traffic-related air pollution and noise: are associations mutually confounded? A systematic review." International journal of public health 58 (2013): 649-666.
46. Goldberg, Mark S., Richard T. Burnett, and Jeffrey R. Brook. "Counterpoint: Time-series studies of acute health events and environmental conditions are not confounded by personal risk factors." Regulatory toxicology and pharmacology 51.2 (2008): 141-147.
47. Hopke, Philip K., Yinchang Feng, Qili Dai, Source apportionment of particle number concentrations: A global review, Science of The Total Environment, Volume 819, 2022
48. Hudda, Neelakshi, et al., "Emissions from an international airport increase particle number concentrations 4-fold at 10 km downwind." Environmental science & technology 48.12 (2014): 6628-6635.

Chapter 6   book Summary and Conclusions

In this last chapter the main findings of the book will be summarized and the significance and novelty of the research discussed. Conclusions and recommendations are provided at the end.

6.1   Main Findings

6.2   Cincinnati study

In the Cincinnati study (book Chapter 2), we found that personal-scale, microenvironmental exposure measurement with novel, wearable sensors is feasible for assessment and evaluation of co-exposures of UFP and noise on health outcomes (heart-rate). We determined that both the highest UFP concentrations and dBA levels which one study participant was jointly exposed to occurred during transit (travelling within a car, truck or bus), and the lowest UFP concentrations and noise levels occurred concurrently while the participant was in other microenvironments (including indoor settings). We also found that measurement of real-time microenvironmental temperature using a wearable sensor provides an accurate measurement ($\sim$ +/-5 degrees F) of ambient microenvironmental temperature, which is useful for understanding UFP and temperature collinearity.

Transportation-related air pollution (TRAP) was measured successfully in real time using a PUFP C200 wearable sampler as particle number concentration (# particles/cc). This serves as a proxy for UFP exposure. UFP measurements were collected concurrently with noise exposure data (dBA) by NEATVIBEwear, a wearable noise monitoring device designed, engineered, and built specifically for this study.

6.3   Greater Boston Studies

In the first Boston study (Chapter 3) of low frequency environmental noise, we found that LFN is predictably present as a component of UEN in the two Environmental Justice communities studied, with statistically significant (*p-vals* <0.05) temporal trends observed. We found that LFN does not follow the same seasonal trends as A-weighted dBA loudness, with Roxbury having higher LAeq levels (dBA) in Spring v. Summer, and Chelsea the reverse, possibly due to disparate community noise and differing seasonal schedules and patterns of transportation sources emitting LFN<125Hz. We also evaluated loudness and noise frequency measures for weeks when school was in-session v. not in-session and found similar trends to seasonality, attributing differences by site to school bus traffic along Roxbury site local roads.

Meteorological covariates (temperature, humidity, barometric pressure, wind speed and direction) were evaluated as predictors of noise outcomes of LAeq and noise frequency dB levels (VLFN, LFN, MFN and HFN). The most significant effect of these meteorological covariates was high wind speeds effects on VLFN, with a substantial increase (β = 12.5; 95% CI: 12.49, 12.58) in VLFN dB levels during high wind speeds at Chelsea, irrespective of wind direction, and to a lesser degree (β = 3.1; 95% CI: 3.11, 3.16) at Roxbury. LFN was minimally affected by high wind speeds at either site. These findings informed our multivariate regression model building in Chapter 5 of this book.

In Chapter 4, a Scalable Machine Learning Approach to Classifying Transportation Noise at Two Urban sites in Greater Boston, Massachusetts, we produced models of transport-associated noise events with varying degrees of accuracy. We randomly selected 60% of our dataset to train and took the remaining 40% to test the model. For binary classifications, we found that the Resnet34 model performed better vs. the 4-layer CNN model; log scale spectrograms produced better accuracy vs. linear scale, and the majority of images were classified correctly. The predicted class for rail (vs. no rail) was 32%. For multi-category classification, we found that log scale maintains relative higher accuracy (71% overall accuracy), and the Resnet34 model produced a better overall fit. The model confusion matrix showed high accuracy for rail (27.8%) and bus (20.8%) classes, but poor classification for airplane noise events (1.4%).

In Chapter 5, our second Boston study, we modeled the association of environmental noise (loudness and frequencies) with ultrafine particles (UFP<100nm diameter), moderated by meteorological factors and site. Our objectives were to establish whether loudness and noise frequencies emitted from urban noise sources identified by metrics such as 1/3-octave band spectral analysis are associated with statistically significant variations in ln(UFP) concentrations, controlling for meteorology, time of day and site; and to determine if effect modification of the noise-UFP association moderated by impact sector wind parameters (i.e. from direction and sources of transportation noise – airport, roadways, rail lines, bus station) has statistically significant associations with elevated ln(UFP) at receptor sites compared to non-impact sector winds.

Based on results of multivariate regression modeling, we developed a wind-robust model based on associations of various low frequency noise components (f<125 Hz), which are also linked to diesel-emitting transportation sources and modeled these noise frequency's interaction with wind speed (km/hr), a significant factor in UFP transport from source to receptor. Our proposed wind-robust models were validated by local work from Hudda et al. (2016), who found that the annual (2014) average impact-sector PNC from Logan Airport was 2-fold higher than the average for all other wind directions, and further supported by Simon et al. (2017) who found that during SSE winds at Chelsea, average PNC was approximately twice the average for all other wind directions. We found similar results. For median values of VLFN (dB), LFN (dB) and wind speed (km/hr) our wind-robust model predicted 21,547 particles/cm^3 from the airport wind impact sector (both sites) and 12,281 particles/cm^3 from impact sector winds from local roads (both sites).

6.4   Significance

To our knowledge, the Chelsea and Roxbury study is one of the longer-term data collection campaigns in which both noise and UFP were continuously sampled. Many transportation noise and PM/UFP studies have focused on evaluating near-highway or urban core receptor impacts from noise (typically as dBA) and PM/UFP based on short durations of data collection of several days to < 1 month. Our data were collected over a five month period ($n = 150$ days) and encompassed co-located noise and PNC measurements.

We identified noise metrics more suitable for urban environmental noise classification than the commonly used and regulated A-weighted (dBA) loudness measures, linking very low frequency noise (VLFN<20Hz) and low frequency noise (LFN: 20 -125Hz) to diesel engine vehicles as a transportation source of importance for their contributory exposure effects of noise and UFP emissions.

The innovation of our approach lies in the identification of noise sources by vehicle class (i.e. heavy trucks, buses or other diesel utility vehicles), as suggested by Chapter 4, and identifying vehicles' dominant noise frequencies and correlating this with the corresponding real-time measurement of PNC as an indicator of UFP exposure, as demonstrated by proxy in Chapter 5.

The Cincinnati study is the first of its kind to utilize personal, real-time exposure measurement of both UFP and noise obtained through the use of wearable sensors. Data sets from the study will facilitate assessment of the impact of short-term and peak exposures on heart rate and other health-based outcomes from co-exposures to UFP and noise.

## 6.5	Recommendations

We recommend disseminating results of this book to the City of Boston in support of adding environmental noise to the list of 15 determinants that influence the health of Boston residents and communities. We also recommend making the large noise dataset (5-months) encompassing 1×10^9 readings available for future research.

Future work is planned to improve machine learning classification rates and publish findings of that study. Lastly, we recommend that our proposed wind robust noise-PNC model, presented in Chapter 5, "Meteorological and Spatiotemporal Associations of Urban Environmental Noise Frequencies with PNC" be replicated in other locations for assessment of the model's generalizability. Possible locations could be those in which we have active collaborations, such as Cincinnati, OH, where the author has previously collaborated with researchers conducting a joint noise and UFP personal exposure study (*Leaffer, et al., 2019*). We also recommend replicating our wind robust model in Los Angeles, CA where one of our Tufts University collaborators conducted a study on long-range (10 km downwind) effects of PNC emissions from aviation emissions (*Hudda, N. et al. 2014*). Historical noise data from the airport may be useful in such a study.

6.6   Conclusions

This book explores the link between chronic, combined exposure to transportation-related noise and ultrafine particle (UFP, <100nm diameter) emissions. Therse joint exposures pose a critical but understudied health risk. This book aims to refine predictive models by concurrently measuring noise and air pollution, enhancing the understanding of their combined health effects.

At the onset of the study, methodologies were developed to encompass measurement, visualization, and analysis of transportation noise measures (frequency, acoustic power, and spectra) concurrently with UFP concentrations. The study goals were to better understand the spatiotemporal variations of noise and UFP, assessing their correlation with meteorological parameters, and to jointly measure personal exposure to noise and UFP in various micro-environments. This book also introduces new health-focused noise metrics, challenging the commonly used occupational standard (dBA) metrics. It explores the link between these metrics and ultrafine particle (UFP) concentrations, studying how noise and air pollution interact under various meteorological conditions.

In our field study conducted in Cincinnati (book Chapter 2) we deployed personal sensors for real-time monitoring of UFP and noise across microenvironments (transit, home, school) and examined their effects on adolescent heart rates. The study further demonstrated the feasibility and relative ease of adding real-time ambient temperature measurements to the personal monitoring sensor platforms. Most exposure studies utilize average daily temperature values from fixed site meteorological records as a proxy for actual exposures, which may vary considerably as participants move between microenvironments. The data collected in this field study will inform future personal-scale exposure assessment studies of similar design.

In the first of our Boston studies (book Chapter 3), we evaluated and recommended alternative noise exposure metrics based on noise frequencies (Hz). Our work advocates for their robust utilization in health-based noise exposure studies, challenging the prevalent dependence on conventional A-weighted decibel (dBA) loudness metrics.

Chapter 4 introduces a scalable machine learning approach for classifying transportation noise by vehicle class, laying the foundation for potential future utilization of machine learning in source identification. The type of machine learning we utilized is classification of patterns of sound. In this approach, we employed transfer learning - using existing models based on thousands of input data files, and we added this to our spectrograms generated from the Boston study data. Transfer learning models find similarities in datasets. Our model was trained on spectrograms, which contain decibels, frequencies and Doppler effects, for image recognition of trucks, trains, and airplanes. Our model can help subclassify other transportation noise source features for future research.

Lastly, our second Boston study (book Chapter 5) utilized multivariate regression to study how noise and ultrafine particles vary with meteorological conditions. It presents and validates a wind-robust model, associating low-frequency noise (<125 Hz) and UFP, factoring in the impact of wind speed on UFP transport. Our proposed wind-robust model, controlling for wind impact sector (direction) has good agreement with prior work conducted at the same sites and may be valid to predict average or median PNC values, based on median noise measures of VLFN (dB) and LFN (dB), with interactions of LFN and median wind speeds. The proposed model may not be as strong a predictor for individual noise-UFP events such as UFP emissions from single components of road traffic (e.g. buses, trucks). The novelty of our wind-robust model is its use of lower noise frequencies as transportation-source proxies, interacting with wind speed to estimate UFP concentrations from impact sector wind directions.

On the whole, this book relies on frequency (f, Hz) as a proxy for tranportation noise source, with diesel-emitting sources linked to frequencies <125Hz. The large dataset in this study is currently being tested for implementing a more robust machine-learning modeling classification approach, which will help further define spatiotemporal differences in both loudness and noise frequencies classified by source (e.g. truck, bus, rail, aircraft). Transportation noise sources identified by machine-learning will be input into regression models with UFP as the outcome, also factoring in effect modifications of wind. It is the expectation that such models will improve understanding of the complex correlations between noise and particulate matter exposure and add significant value to the quality of air pollution models.

Appendix 1. Supplementary Materials for Chapter 3

Appendix 2. Supplementary Materials for Chapter 5

Table 5S

Model	Independent Variables	Intercept ln(UFP) ~1	Effect Estimate (95% ci)	Adjusted R^2	RMSE	p-val	AIC
Model 1 (C2)		10.1	(9.9, 10.2)	0.30	0.60		1.99e+05
moise, weather	LAeq (dBA)		0.007 (0.005, 0.009)			<0.001	
and spatiotemporal	VLFN (<20 Hz)		-0.020 (-0.021, -0.019)			0	
factors)	Day_1 (0700-2300HRS)		0.20 (0.19, 0.21)			0	
	Site_1		-3.5 (-3.6, -3.3)			0	
	Temp(°C)		-0.004 (-0.005, -0.003)			<0.001	
Interactions:	Humidity (%)		-0.003 (-0.004, -0.002)			<0.001	
(Site_0==Chelsea	Site_1:LAeq		0.028 (0.024, 0.03)			<0.001	
Site_1==Roxbury)	Site_1:VLFN		0.039 (0.038, 0.04)			0	
Model 2 (F2)		9.44	(9.33, 9.56)	0.34	0.59		1.88e+05
moise, weather	VLFN (<20 Hz)		-0.0021 (-0.022, -0.02)			0	
and spatiotemporal	LFN(20 -125 Hz)		0.016 (0.014, 0.018)			<0.001	
factors)	Day_1 (0700-2300HRS)		0.12 (0.11, 0.13)			<0.001	
	Site_1		-5.0 (-5.1, -4.8)			0	
	Temp(°C)		-0.006 (-0.007, -0.005)			<0.001	
Interactions:	Humidity (%)		-0.0025(-0.003,-0.002)			<0.001	
(Site_0==Chelsea	Site_1:VLFN		0.01 (0.008, 0.011)			<0.001	
Site_1==Roxbury	Site_1:LFN		0.07 (0.066, 0.08)			0	
Model 3 (36ee)		9.56	(9.4, 9.7)	0.33	0.59		1.40e+05
(Wind Speed =LO	LAeq (dBA)		0.02 (0.018, 0.022)			<0.001	
effect modifications)	VLFN (<20 Hz)		-0.022 (-0.023, -0.021)			0	
	Day_1 (0700-2300HRS)		0.13 (0.12, 0.14)			<0.001	
	Site_1		-3.6 (-3.8, -3.4)			0	
	Temp(°C)		-0.008 (-0.009, -0.007)			<0.001	
Interactions:	Humidity (%)		-0.003(-.0033,-.0028)			<0.001	
(Site_0==Chelsea	Site_1:LAeq		-0.007 (-0.01,- 0.0036)			<0.001	
Site_1==Roxbury)	Site_1:VLFN		0.074 (0.073, 0.075)			0	
Model 4 (31ee)		11.3	(11.1, 11.5)	0.34	0.57		4.79+04
(Wind Speed =HI	LAeq (dBA)		-0.021 (-0.027, -0.02)			<0.001	
effect modifications)	VLFN (<20 Hz)		-0.016 (-0.017, -0.014)			<0.001	
	Day_1 (0700-2300HRS)		0.35 (0.33, 0.37)			<0.001	
	Site_1		-4.5 (-4.8, -4.1)			<0.001	
	Temp(°C)		0.002 (0.0012, 0.003)			<0.001	
Interactions:	Humidity (%)		-0.005(-.0052,-.0045)			<0.001	
(Site_0==Chelsea	Site_1:LAeq		0.07 (0.064, 0.075)			<0.001	
Site_1==Roxbury	Site_1:VLFN		0.014 (0.011, 0.017)			<0.001	
Model 5 (38ee)		9.14	(9.01, 9.28)	0.34	0.58		1.38e+05
(Wind Speed =LO	VLFN (<20 Hz)		-0.0021 (-0.022, -0.02)			<0.001	
effect modifications)	LFN(20 -125 Hz)		0.022 (0.019, 0.024)			<0.001	
	Day_1 (0700-2300HRS)		0.09 (0.08, 0.10)			<0.001	
	Site_1		-5.0 (-5.19, -4.83)			0	
	Temp(°C)		-0.008 (-0.009, -0.007)			<0.001	
Interactions:	Humidity (%)		-0.0026(-0.003,-0.002)			<0.001	
(Site_0==Chelsea	Site_1:VLFN		0.042 (0.039, 0.044)			<0.001	
Site_1==Roxbury	Site_1:LFN		0.042 (0.039, 0.045)			<0.001	
Model 6 (33ee)		10.2	(9.98, 10.4)	0.38	0.55		4.61e+04
(Wind Speed =HI	VLFN (<20 Hz)		-0.018 (-0.02, -0.016)			<0.001	
effect modifications)	LFN(20 -125 Hz)		0.002 (-0.0017, 0.006)			0.28*	
	Day_1 (0700-2300HRS)		0.18 (0.16, 0.20)			<0.001	
	Site_1		-5.8 (-6.16, -5.5)			<0.001	
	Temp(°C)		-0.003 (-0.004, -0.002)			<0.001	
Interactions:	Humidity (%)		-0.0046(-0.005,-0.004)			<0.001	
(Site_0==Chelsea	Site_1:VLFN		-0.0004(-0.003, 0.002)			0.80*	
Site_1==Roxbury	Site_1:LFN		0.089 (0.084, 0.094)			<0.001	
* p-val >0.05							

Model	Independent Variables	Intercept ln(UFP) ~1	Effect Estimate (95% ci)	Adjusted R^2	RMSE	p-val	AIC
Model 7 (N)		9.64	(9.54, 9.74)	0.124	0.584		7.18+04
Site==Chelsea	L.Aeq (dBA)		0.0085 (0.007, 0.01)			<0.001	
	VLFN(<20 Hz)		-0.019 (-0.02, -0.018)			0	
	Day (0700 -2300HRS)		0.176 (0.161, 0.190)			<0.001	
Interactions *(Noise and Wind Impact Sectors)*	L.Aeq:Impact Wind_rail		-0.028 (-0.03, -0.02)			<0.001	
	L.Aeq:Wind_airport		0.013 (0.007, 0.018)			<0.001	
	L.Aeq:Impact_Wind_road		-0.008 (-0.01, -0.056)			<0.001	
	VLFN:Impact Wind_rail		0.019 (0.017, 0.021)			<0.001	
	VLFN:Wind_airport		-0.006 (-0.01, -.0012)			0.014	
	VLFN:Impact_Wind_road		-0.012 (0.01, 0.015)			<0.001	
Model 8 (O)		9.35	(9.24, 9.47)	0.125	0.583		7.17+04
Site==Chelsea	VLFN(<20 Hz)		-0.02 (0.021, -0.01)			<0.001	
	LFN (20 – 125 Hz)		0.012 (0.010, 0.014)			<0.001	
	Day (0700 -2300HRS)		0.167 (0.153, 0.181)			<0.001	
Interactions *(Noise and Wind Impact Sectors)*	VLFN:Impact Wind_rail		0.022 (0.020, 0.025)			<0.001	
	VLFN:Wind_airport		-0.017 (-0.02, -0.012)			<0.001	
	VLFN:Impact_Wind_road		0.012 (0.01, 0.015)			<0.001	
	LFN:Impact Wind_rail		-0.026 (-0.09, -0.024)			<0.001	
	LFN:Wind_airport		0.020 (0.015, 0.025)			<0.001	
	LFN:Impact_Wind_road		-0.007 (-0.01, -0.005)			<0.001	
Model 9 (V)		6.32	(6.19, 6.46)	0.149	0.59		1.17+05
Site==Roxbury	L.Aeq (dBA)		0.033 (0.031, 0.036)			<0.001	
	VLFN(<20 Hz)		0.017 (0.016, 0.019)			<0.001	
	Day (0700 -2300HRS)		0.28 (0.269, 0.293)			0	
Interactions *(Noise and Wind Impact Sectors)*	L.Aeq:Wind_airport		0.011 (0.005, 0.017)			0.0002	
	L.Aeq:Impact_Wind_road		-0.012 (-0.02, -0.006)			<0.001	
	L.Aeq:Impact_Wind_bus		0.015 (0.01, 0.02)			<0.001	
	VLFN:Wind_airport		-0.006 (-0.01, 0.001)			0.086*	
	VLFN:Impact_Wind_road		0.013 (0.008, 0.019)			<0.001	
	VLFN:Impact_Wind_bus		-0.014 (-0.02, -0.01)			<0.001	
Model 10 (X)		4.05	(3.91, 4.19)	0.218	0.57		1.12+05
Site==Roxbury	L.Aeq (dBA)		0.077 (0.075, 0.079)			0	
	LFN(20 -125 Hz)		-0.0005 (-.003, .002)			0.693*	
	Day (0700 -2300HRS)		0.113 (0.102, 0.125)			<0.001	
Interactions *(Noise and Wind Impact Sectors)*	L.Aeq:Wind_airport		-0.01 (-0.02, -0.0005)			0.038	
	L.Aeq:Impact_Wind_road		0.014 (0.007, 0.022)			<0.001	
	L.Aeq:Impact_Wind_bus		-0.04 (0.05, -0.09)			<0.001	
	LFN:Wind_airport		0.013 (0.005, 0.02)			0.001	
	LFN:Impact_Wind_road		-0.01 (-0.017, -0.004)			<0.001	
	LFN:Impact_Wind_bus		0.034 (0.027, 0.041)			<0.001	

*p-val >0.05

Supplementary autocorrelation lag-time plots for Chapter 5 Noise Measures

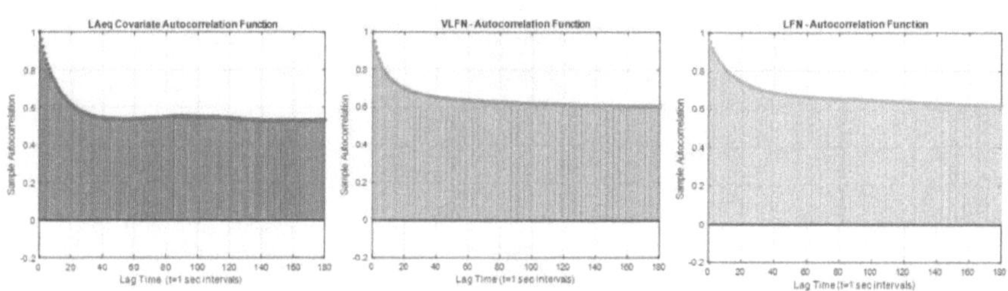

Supplementary Tables for Chapter 5

Table S6

Supplemental Ch. 5

Note: Airport and Road wind impact sectors are common to both Sites

Wind Robust Model
Eq(1): ln(UFP) ~ βo + β1*VLFN (dB) + β2*LFN (dB) + β3*[LFN*(wind_speed (km/hr)] + e

Impact_Wind_Airport (both Sites; n=5000 observations)

mdl_WR2	estimate	SE	tStat	pval
Intercept	3.289713	0.167285	19.6653	5.49E-83
VLFN	-0.02769	0.00247	-11.2108	7.95E-29
LFN	0.119287	0.002978	40.05884	1.5E-304
LFN:WS	-0.00011	2.27E-05	-4.99422	6.11E-07
AIC =	9614.414	Rsquared	0.273	

PNC Prediction = 19270.42 #/cm^3

*Median noise and wind measures

VLFN	62.733 dB
LFN	70.565 dB
MFN	59.458 dB
LAeq(t=1n	58.8 dBA
wind sp.	12.964 km/hr

* combined sites for airport WD

Wind Robust Model   dBA
ln(UFP) ~ βo + β1*LAeq (dBA) + e

Impact_Wind_Airport Roxbury only; n= observations)

mdl_WR2	estimate	SE	tStat	pval
Intercept	5.659454	0.135636	41.72537	0
LAeq(t=1n	0.071256	0.002327	30.61754	7.8E-189
AIC =	10346.9	Rsquared	0.158	

PNC Predicton = 18945.5 #/cm^3

Wind Robust Model
Eq(1): ln(UFP) ~ βo + β1*VLFN (dB) + β2*LFN (dB) + β3*[LFN*(wind_speed (km/hr)] + e

Impact_Wind_Road (both Sites; n=11515 observations)

mdl_WR8	estimate	SE	tStat	pval
Intercept	5.478947	0.091621	59.79991	0
VLFN	-0.01216	0.000941	-12.9241	6.04E-38
LFN	0.071809	0.001276	56.28507	0
LFN:WS	-0.00016	1.18E-05	-13.2942	4.93E-40
AIC =	17735.29	Rsquared	0.217	

PNC Prediction = 14512.25 #/cm^3

*Median noise and wind measures

VLFN	64.216 dB
LFN	70.591 dB
MFN	59.243 dB
LAeq(t=1n	58.2 dBA
wind sp.	16.668 km/hr

* combined sites for roadway WD

Wind Robust Model   dBA
ln(UFP) ~ βo + β1*LAeq (dBA) + e

Impact_Wind_Road (both Sites; n=11515 observations)

mdl_WR8	estimate	SE	tStat	pval
Intercept	6.321092	0.072253	87.48606	0
LAeq(t=1n	0.056023	0.001251	44.76811	0
AIC =	18708.59	Rsquared	0.148	

PNC Prediction = 14495.64 #/cm^3

Wind Robust Model   deltaC-A + WS
ln(UFP) ~ βo + β1*deltaC-A (dB) + β2*[deltaC-A*(wind_speed (km/hr)] + e
both Sites; n=200 observations; all wind directions

mdl_WR2	estimate	SE	tStat	pval
Intercept	10.61052	0.286503	37.03459	1.96E-90
deltaC-A	-0.12277	0.029451	-4.16861	4.6E-05
deltaC-A:\	0.000269	0.000514	0.523776	0.601026
AIC =	315.6	Rsquared	0.073	pval>0.05

PNC Predicton   11882.56 #/cm^3
median deltaC-A = 9.96 dB (use 10 dB in models)
median daily WS = 11.11 km/hr
NOTE: PNC increases as deltaC-A decreases here

Wind Robust Model   deltaC-A + ImpactWind
ln(UFP) ~ βo + β1*deltaC-A (dB) + β2*[deltaC-A*(ImpactWind] + e
both Sites; n=200 observations; wind speed removed

mdl_WR2	estimate	SE	tStat	pval
Intercept	10.28481	0.26984	38.11453	9.19E-92
deltaC-A	-0.0808	0.027315	-2.95814	0.003482
deltaC-A:r	-0.09429	0.019019	-4.9578	1.56E-06
deltaC-A:a	-0.041	0.018147	-2.2595	0.02497
deltaC-A:r	-0.03452	0.011722	-2.94454	0.003632
deltaC-A:l	0.037714	0.016633	2.267496	0.024468
AIC =	282.8	Rsquared	0.226	

PNC Predi	rail	13052.5 #/cm^3
PNC Predi	airport	13053.03 #/cm^3
PNC Predi	road	13053.1 #/cm^3
PNC Predi	bus-sta	13053.82 #/cm^3

Wind Robust Model   dBA + WS
ln(UFP) ~ βo + β1*LAeq (dBA)+ β2*[LAeq*(wind_speed (km/hr)]

Impact_Wind_Airport (both Sites; n=5000 observations)

mdl_WR2t	estimate	SE	tStat	pval
Intercept	5.457797	0.1417	38.51655	2E-284
LAeq(t=1n	0.076615	0.002576	29.73825	4.5E-179
LAeq:WS	-0.00013	2.66E-05	-4.80307	1.61E-06
AIC =	10325.87	Rsquared	0.1615	

PNC Prediction =   19252.02 #/cm^3

Wind Robust Model   dBA + WS
ln(UFP) ~ βo + β1*LAeq (dBA)+ β2*[LAeq*(wind_speed (km/hr)]
Impact_Wind_Road (both Sites; n=11515 observations)

mdl_WR2t	estimate	SE	tStat	pval
Intercept	5.457797	0.1417	38.51655	2E-284
LAeq(t=1n	0.076615	0.002576	29.73825	4.5E-179
LAeq:WS	-0.00013	2.66E-05	-4.80307	1.61E-06
AIC =	10325.87	Rsquared	0.1615	

PNC Prediction =   20268.11 #/cm^3

Wind Robust Model   dBA + deltaC-A +WS
ln(UFP) ~ βo + β1*LAeq (dBA) + β2*deltaC-A (dB) + e
both Sites; n=200 observations; all wind directions

mdl_WR2(	estimate	SE	tStat	pval
Intercept	0.053776	1.108626	0.048507	0.961362
LAeq(t=1d	0.164875	0.01813	9.093894	1.14E-16
deltaC-A	-0.03085	0.038264	-0.80636	0.421021
LAeq:WS	-7.5E-05	0.000526	-0.14226	0.887021
deltaC-A:\	0.000657	0.00299	0.2197	0.826336
AIC =	239.7396	Rsquared	0.373	pval>0.05

PNC Predicton   13316.4 #/cm^3
median deltaC-A = 9.96 dB (use 10 dB in models)
median daily WS = 11.11 km/hr
median LAeq(1-day)   59 dBA

Wind Robust Model   dBA + VLFN
ln(UFP) ~ βo + β1*LAeq (dBA)+ β2*VLFN + e

Impact_Wind_Airport (both Sites; n=5000 observations)

mdl_WR2	estimate	SE	tStat	pval
Intercept	5.722293	0.144631	39.56469	4.5E-298
LAeq(t=1n	0.07249	0.002742	26.43341	3.1E-144
VLFN	-0.00215	0.002168	-0.99351	0.320509
AIC =	10356.37	Rsquared	0.157	

PNC Prediction =   21691.74 #/cm^3

Wind Robust Model   dBA + VLFN
ln(UFP) ~ βo + β1*LAeq (dBA)+ β2*VLFN + e
Impact_Wind_Road (both Sites; n=11559 observations)

mdl_WR2	estimate	SE	tStat	pval
Intercept	6.85899	0.080712	84.98146	0
LAeq(t=1n	0.060741	0.001279	47.47857	0
VLFN	-0.01255	0.000866	-14.489	3.68E-47
AIC =	18557.02	Rsquared	0.164	

PNC Prediction =   32665.2 #/cm^3

Wind Robust Model ROXBURY dBA
ln(UFP) ~ βo + β1*LAeq (dBA) + e
Impact_Wind_Airport (Roxbury; n=3497 observations)

mdl_ROX_	estimate	SE	tStat	pval
Intercept	4.586906	0.278839	16.45002	1.27E-58
LAeq(t=1n	0.089948	0.004634	19.40972	8.78E-80
AIC =	7137.5	Rsquared	0.097	

PNC Predicton   21672.56 #/cm^3
median LAeq(1-min)   60 dBA

Wind Robust Model ROXBURY dBA + VLFN +LFN
ln(UFP) ~ βo + β1*LAeq (dBA)+ β2*VLFN + β3*LFN + ε
Impact_Wind_Airport (Roxbury; n=3497 observations

mdl_ROX_	estimate	SE	tStat
Intercept	2.072595	0.278789	7.434266
LAeq(t=1n	0.001827	0.005769	0.31673
VLFN	-0.0214	0.003697	-5.78946
LFN	0.127769	0.005708	22.38342
AIC =	6605.913	Rsquared	0.225

PNC Predicton   22959.81 #/cm^3
median LAeq(1-min)   60 dBA
median VLFN (dB) =   63.721 dB
median LFN (dB) =   72.186 dB

Wind Robust Model ROXBURY dBA

ln(UFP) ~ βo + β1*LAeq (dBA) + e

Impact_Wind_Other (Roxbury; n=52919 observations)

mdl_ROX_	estimate	SE	tStat	pval	
Intercept	5.513779	0.069734	79.06922		0
LAeq(t=1m	0.068948	0.00116	59.4311		0
AIC =		97291.56	Rsquared	0.063	

PNC Predicton	15585.25 #/cm^3
median LAeq(1-min)	60.05 dBA

Wind Robust Model ROXBURY dBA + VLFN +LFN

ln(UFP) ~ βo + β1*LAeq (dBA)+ β2*VLFN + β3*LFN + e

Impact_Wind_Other (Roxbury; n=52919 observations

mdl_ROX_	estimate	SE	tStat
Intercept	3.450559	0.068881	50.09438
LAeq(t=1m	-0.00092	0.00133	-0.69148
VLFN	-0.00408	0.000819	-4.9834
LFN	0.090693	0.001202	75.42957
AIC =	89549.27	Rsquared	0.19

PNC Predicton	16098.18 #/cm^3
median LAeq(1-min)	60.05 dBA
median VLFN (dB) =	63.33 dB
median LFN (dB) =	72.216 dB

Wind Robust Model

Eq(1):   ln(UFP) ~ βo + β1*LFN (dB)

Impact_Wind_Road (both Sites; n=10996 observations)

mdl_CRrd	estimate	SE	tStat	pval	
Intercept	5.598918	0.082602	67.78163		0
LFN	0.056073	0.001181	47.4984		0
AIC =		16116	Rsquared	0.17	

PNC Prediction =   13996.41 #/cm^3

*Median noise and wind measures

VLFN	64.196 dB
LFN	70.402 dB
MFN	59.243 dB
WS	16.668 km/hr
LAeq(t=1m	58.2 dBA

* combined sites for roadway WD

Wind Robust Model

Eq(1):   ln(UFP) ~ βo + β1*LFN (dB) + β2*WS (km/hr)

Impact_Wind_Road (both Sites; n=10996 observations)

mdl_CRrd	estimate	SE	tStat	pval
Intercept	5.5833	0.081549	68.46553	0
LFN	0.059165	0.00118	50.15928	0
WS	-0.01256	0.00074	-16.9779	7.77E-64
AIC =	15833.38	Rsquared	0.1913	

Confounding Check

	β (no WS)	β (with WS	%diff.
VLFN	0.056073	0.059165	0.053662

Wind Robust Model
Eq(1):   ln(UFP) ~ βo + β1*VLFN (dB)

Impact_Wind_Airport (both Sites; n=3920 observations)

mdl_CRai	estimate	SE	tStat	pval
Intercept	8.886404	0.105918	83.89882	0
VLFN	0.013507	0.001702	7.93479	2.73E-15
AIC =	6964.762	Rsquared	0.0156	

PNC Prediction =   16877.28 #/cm^3

Wind Robust Model
Eq(1):   ln(UFP) ~ βo + β1*VLFN (dB) WS (km/hr)

Impact_Wind_Airport (both Sites; n=3920 observations)

mdl_CRai	estimate	SE	tStat	pval
Intercept	9.057569	0.113016	80.14403	0
VLFN	0.009104	0.001986	4.583218	4.72E-06
WS	0.007259	0.001698	4.274796	1.96E-05
AIC =	6966.517	Rsquared	0.0199	

PNC Prediction =   16693.82 #/cm^3

Confounding Check

	β (no WS)	β (with WS)	%diff.
VLFN	0.013507	0.009104	0.389447

Wind Robust Model
Eq(1):   ln(UFP) ~ βo + β1*LFN (dB)

Impact_Wind_Airport (both Sites; n=3920 observations)

mdl_CRai	estimate	SE	tStat	pval
Intercept	5.423499	0.142157	38.1514	4.2E-271
LFN	0.061782	0.002039	30.30307	2.1E-181
AIC =	6221.844	Rsquared	0.189	

PNC Prediction =   10930.01 #/cm^3

Wind Robust Model
Eq(1):   ln(UFP) ~ βo + β1*LFN (dB) +β2*WS (km/hr)

Impact_Wind_Airport (both Sites; n=3920 observations)

mdl_CRai	estimate	SE	tStat	pval
Intercept	5.260658	0.147901	35.56887	2.2E-240
LFN	0.065252	0.002221	29.38389	1.1E-171
WS	-0.00562	0.001438	-3.9048	9.59E-05
AIC =	6968.517	Rsquared	0.0199	

PNC Prediction =   17896.73 #/cm^3

Confounding Check

	β (no WS)	β (with WS)	%diff.
LFN	0.061782	0.065252	0.054633

Wind Robust Model   dBA
ln(UFP) ~ βo + β1*LAeq (dBA) + e

Impact_Wind_Airport Roxbury only; n= observations)

mdl_WR2i	estimate	SE	tStat	pval
Intercept	5.659454	0.135636	41.72537	0
LAeq(t=1n	0.071256	0.002327	30.61754	7.8E-189
AIC =	10346.9	Rsquared	0.158	

Confounding Check

	β (no WS)	β (with WS)	%diff.
dBA	0.071256	-0.00013	2.007188

Wind Robust Model   dBA + WS
ln(UFP) ~ βo + β1*LAeq (dBA)+ β2*[LAeq*(wind_speed)] + e

Impact_Wind_Airport (both Sites; n=5000 observations)

mdl_WR2t	estimate	SE	tStat	pval
Intercept	5.457797	0.1417	38.51655	2E-284
LAeq(t=1n	0.076815	0.002576	29.73825	4.5E-179
LAeq:WS	-0.00013	2.66E-05	-4.80307	1.61E-06
AIC =	10325.87	Rsquared	0.1615	

Wind Robust Model
Eq(1):   ln(UFP) ~ βo + β1*VLFN (dB) + β2*LFN (dB)

Impact_Wind_Airport (both Sites; n=3920 observations)

mdl_CRai	estimate	SE	tStat	pval
Intercept	5.445896	0.137822	39.51393	1.1E-287
VLFN	-0.03188	0.002009	-15.8678	5.29E-55
LFN	0.089851	0.002652	33.87416	7.9E-221
AIC =	5979.631	Rsquared	0.238	

PNC Prediction =   17785.41 #/cm^3

*Median noise and wind measures

VLFN	62.733 dB
LFN	70.565 dB
MFN	59.458 dB
LAeq(t=1n	58.8 dBA
wind sp.	12.964 km/hr

* combined sites for airport WD

Wind Robust Model
Eq(1):   ln(UFP) ~ βo + β1*VLFN (dB) + β2*LFN (dB) + WS (km/hr)

Impact_Wind_Airport (both Sites; n=3920 observations)

mdl_CRai	estimate	SE	tStat	pval
Intercept	5.532598	0.144661	38.24518	3.2E-272
VLFN	-0.03345	0.002161	-15.4809	1.63E-52
LFN	0.089404	0.002661	33.59504	1.2E-217
WS	0.002952	0.001502	1.965519	0.049425
AIC =	5977.765	Rsquared	0.239	

PNC Prediction =   17701.93 #/cm^3

Confounding Check

	β (no WS)	β (with WS)	%diff.
VLFN	-0.03188	-0.03345	-0.0479
LFN	0.089851	0.089404	0.004982

Wind Robust Model
Eq(1):   ln(UFP) ~ βo + β1*VLFN (dB) + β2*LFN (dB)

Impact_Wind_Road (both Sites; n=10996 observations)

mdl_CRrd	estimate	SE	tStat	pval
Intercept	6.095208	0.085017	71.69374	0
VLFN	-0.01609	0.000818	-19.6747	1.01E-84
LFN	0.063839	0.001226	52.06682	0
AIC =	15737.46	Rsquared	0.1983	

PNC Prediction =   14306.42 #/cm^3

*Median noise and wind measures

VLFN	64.216 dB
LFN	70.581 dB
MFN	59.243 dB
LAeq(t=1n	58.2 dBA

* combined sites for roadway WD

Wind Robust Model
Eq(1):   ln(UFP) ~ βo + β1*VLFN (dB) + β2*LFN (dB) + β3*WS (km/hr)

Impact_Wind_Road (both Sites; n=10996 observations)

mdl_CRrd	estimate	SE	tStat	pval
Intercept	5.97269	0.085578	69.79203	0
VLFN	-0.01243	0.000896	-13.8774	2.02E-43
LFN	0.064016	0.001221	52.44955	0
WS	-0.00789	0.000807	-9.76913	1.88E-22
AIC =	15644.4	Rsquared	0.205	

PNC Prediction =   14630.8 #/cm^3

Confounding Check

	β (no WS)	β (with WS)	%diff.
VLFN	-0.01609	-0.01243	-0.25621
LFN	0.063839	0.064016	0.002774

Wind Robust Model
Eq(1):   ln(UFP) ~ βo + β1*VLFN (dB)

mdl_CRrd	estimate	SE	tStat	pval
Intercept	9.668868	0.056057	172.4831	0
VLFN	-0.00237	0.000864	-2.74377	0.006064
AIC =	18160.93	Rsquared	0.000593	

PNC Prediction =   13583.77 #/cm^3

VLFN	64.196 dB
LFN	70.402 dB
MFN	59.243 dB
WS	16.668 km/hr
LAeq(t=1n	58.2 dBA

* combined sites for roadway WD

Wind Robust Model
Eq(1):   ln(UFP) ~ βo + β1*VLFN (dB) + β2*WS (km/hr)

Impact_Wind_Road (both Sites; n=10996 observations)

mdl_CRrd	estimate	SE	tStat	pval
Intercept	9.565284	0.057361	166.7548	0
VLFN	0.001026	0.00096	1.068417	0.285356
WS	-0.00726	0.000902	-8.04058	9.86E-16
AIC =	18098.45	Rsquared	0.006346	

PNC Prediction =   13496.5 #/cm^3

Confounding Check

	β (no WS)	β (with WS)	%diff.
VLFN	-0.00237	0.001026	-5.04745